PSYCHOLOGY FOR NURSES AND THE CARING PROFESSIONS

SOCIAL SCIENCE FOR NURSES AND THE CARING PROFESSIONS

Series Editor: Professor Pamela Abbott
Pro-Vice-Chancellor, Glasgow Caledonian University, Glasgow, Scotland

Current and forthcoming titles

Community Care for Nurses and the Caring Professions
Nigel Malin *et al.*

Epidemiology: An Introduction
Graham Moon, Myles Gould *et al.*

Nursing People in Psychiatric Systems
Chris Stevenson

**Research Methods for Nurses and the Caring Professions
(2nd edn)**
Pamela Abbott and Roger Sapsford

Research into Practice (2nd edn)
Edited by Pamela Abbott and Roger Sapsford

**Social Perspectives on Pregnancy and Childbirth for Midwives,
Nurses and the Caring Professions**
Julie Kent

Social Policy for Nurses and the Caring Professions
Louise Ackers and Pamela Abbott

PSYCHOLOGY FOR NURSES AND THE CARING PROFESSIONS

2nd edition

Jan Walker, Sheila Payne,
Paula Smith and Nikki Jarrett

Open University Press

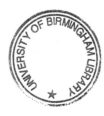

Open University Press
McGraw-Hill Education
McGraw-Hill House
Shoppenhangers Road
Maidenhead
Berkshire
England
SL6 2QL

email: enquiries@openup.co.uk
world wide web: www.openup.co.uk

and Two Penn Plaza, New York, NY 10121-2289, USA

First published 1996. Reprinted 1997, 1998, 1999, 2000, 2001 (twice), 2002

First published in this second edition, 2004 © Jan Walker, Sheila Payne, Paula Smith
and Nikki Jarrett 2004

A catalogue record of this book is available from the British Library

ISBN 0 335 214622 (pb)   0 335 215017 (hb)   22873783

Library of Congress Cataloging-in-Publication Data
CIP data has been applied for

Typeset by RefineCatch Ltd, Bungay, Suffolk
Printed in the UK by Bell & Bain Ltd, Glasgow

CONTENTS

SERIES EDITOR'S PREFACE

It is now widely recognised that the Social Sciences are central to Nurse Education. Nursing as a profession needs to ground itself in an understanding of social structures and social relations, state policies and their constraints on the behaviours and experiences of individuals and groups. The series, of which this is one volume, aims to provide nurses and others in the caring professions with lively and accessible introductions to the issues and debates within the social science disciplines as relevant to their professional practice.

This is the second edition of the very successful *Psychology for Nurses and the Caring Professions* text. The authors are to be congratulated on producing a text that so evidently meets the needs of health care professionals. The book aims to encourage health care professionals in their clinical practice. The authors are all nurses and health psychologists and in writing the text have been able to draw on both their experience of clinical practice and their research interests as psychologists. They are able to use their experience to write an accessible and relevant introduction to psychology that will be used widely by nurses and other caring professionals on pre- and post-registration courses, and will be of relevance to those who have completed their training.

The text not only enables the reader to gain an understanding of the relevance of psychology to nurses and other caring professionals but, more generally, introduces many of the central debates and ideas of psychology, thus providing a general introduction to the discipline. Recognising that the relevance of psychology to clinical practice is not necessarily immediately apparent, the authors explicitly set out to demonstrate the value of psychological understanding to the everyday practice of health care workers. Their aim is not to provide caring professionals with a set of techniques that can be followed in order to improve practice – though psychology is relevant to caring practice – but to introduce them to a way of thinking about individuals and social relationships. The insights that are gained will provide techniques that can be used in professional practice, but more importantly they will enable practitioners to make more sense of the lives of the individuals with whom they are working, and extend the range of ways in which they can help them. Specifically, psychology will help to inform them about vulnerable groups with whom they work – babies, children, older people, people with learning disabilities and those having trouble coping with the strains and demands of contemporary life. It will also provide insights into the problems and difficulties of coping with long-term chronic illness and the complex ways in which habits and attitudes are formed and become resistant to change

Pamela Abbott

PREFACE

The second edition of this book is similar to the first in terms of the intended audience and topics covered, but it has been extensively rewritten to accommodate a number of important changes. While much traditional psychological theory and research remains valid, there have been many advances in psychological knowledge during the past eight years and we have updated the content to reflect these. The inclusion of two new authors has enabled us to cover a wider range of topics in more depth. Paula Smith and Nikki Jarrett are both health psychologists with nursing backgrounds, who teach psychology to health care professionals at this level.

We have responded to the requirement for health care to be evidence-based with the inclusion of many more research examples and references for readers to follow up. However, we have tried not to overload the text with references to material that is widely known and accepted in the public domain. In Chapter 1, we have included a 'psychosoap' family scenario and draw on this periodically throughout the book to illustrate how theory and research can be applied to practice. Many of the situations illustrated are based on actual observations and the scenario used as a convenient way of preserving anonymity. Icons are used in the text to distinguish between scenario 🏃 and research ⚕ extracts. We have included an updated glossary that enables the reader to look up psychological terms that may not be familiar, including words highlighted in **bold** in the text.

In this edition, we present the topics in changed order so that Chapters 7 and 8 on stress, coping, health beliefs and health-related behaviours build on psychological principles presented in earlier chapters. We have omitted the chapter on pain, but have instead included an actual case study to illustrate how health care professionals can use psychological principles from each chapter to contribute to the assessment and management of someone with complex problems including pain. As in the previous edition, we do not address abnormal psychology. All of the psychological issues we have identified draw on psychological theory and research that are applicable to normal populations.

Jan Walker
Sheila Payne
Paula Smith
Nikki Jarrett

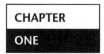

CHAPTER

ONE

WHAT IS PSYCHOLOGY?

KEY

QUESTIONS

- What can psychology contribute to health and health care?
- What is psychology and what are the main approaches to psychological thinking and research?
- Who are psychologists and what do they contribute to the promotion of health and well-being?
- How can we learn to apply psychology to all aspects of health and health care?
- How can psychology help us to explain **anxiety** in real situations?

Introduction

This chapter examines the question 'what is psychology?'. We explore the nature of psychological theories and their relevance to health care. We outline the different schools of thought in psychology and methods of inquiry. We seek to distinguish between psychology as an academic discipline and popular notions of psychology. In order to show how psychology can be applied to health and health care, we introduce a family scenario whose characters will appear throughout the book. We draw on this to illustrate how different schools of psychological thought can provide different interpretations of a common situation. Finally, we identify health care professionals whose practice is mainly concerned with the application of psychology. In reading this chapter, it is important to note that psychology has evolved from western philosophy, science and research and may therefore be viewed as specific to western cultures. This chapter is contextual. It contains material that is drawn largely from secondary sources and is to be found in most undergraduate psychology textbooks. Where necessary, we have referred the reader to sources in other chapters of this book.

What is psychology and why is it important in health care?

Psychology is the study of human behaviour, thought processes and emotions. It can contribute to our understanding of ourselves, and our relationships with other people, if it is applied in an informed way. Those working in the caring professions spend most, if not all, of their working lives interacting with other people. The purpose of this book is to enable practitioners to apply psychology to enhance their therapeutic work, promote the health and well-being of patients (or clients) and carers, preserve their personal sense of well-being, and work more effectively with colleagues in multiprofessional teams.

Psychology must take account of the context of people's lives. Certain sets of beliefs and behaviours are risk factors for illness; therefore some knowledge of public health and the public health agenda for change is essential. Those we care for come from a variety of different social and cultural backgrounds that value certain beliefs and behaviours above others. These may place some people at greater or lesser risk of illness than others; therefore some knowledge of sociology is essential. In order to understand the link between psychological and physiological processes, some knowledge of the biomedical sciences is also essential. The psychology of health cannot be viewed in isolation from these other disciplines.

There are many ways in which psychological theory and research can contribute to improvements in health and social care, including:

- Appreciating how people's comprehension and needs vary, so that we can try to ensure that the individualized care we provide is both appropriate and optimal.
- Gaining a better understanding of communication processes so that we can identify ways of improving the therapeutic relationship and work more effectively in interprofessional and inter-agency contexts.
- Identifying factors that affect how people cope with such situations as acute and chronic illness, pain and loss, and the demands of everyday life, so that we can help them to cope better and reduce the risks of stress-related illness.
- Informing us about factors that influence whether or not people are likely to engage in certain **health-related behaviours** such as smoking, dietary change and exercise, so that we can help them to change or modify their lifestyles in order to enhance their long-term health and well-being.

Different perspectives in psychology

Functioning as a person involves coping with social and psychological aspects of everyday life as well as having fully functioning body systems, but divisions between health-related disciplines have made holistic care difficult. Descartes, a French philosopher in the seventeenth century, proposed that body and mind could be understood independently of each other. This is referred to as mind–body **dualism**. In medical science, this has legitimized the study of body systems without focusing on the whole person. In psychology, the predominance of the study of the mind meant that the individual was often studied in isolation from their social context and social groupings. In the human sciences, divisions have given rise to the separation of the life sciences from the social sciences and the development of a series of unrelated academic disciplines, including physiology, psychology and sociology. Each discipline has its own sets of theories, terminology and research methods with which to study the human condition.

Meanwhile, various health and social care professions have developed independently, each with their own sets of assumptions and theoretical perspectives. These include medicine, physiotherapy, occupational therapy, midwifery and social work, while nursing has been subdivided into adult, child, mental health and learning disability. Each of these disciplines seeks to explain human responses, predict human needs and/or treat human problems. But they often draw on different bodies of knowledge which sometimes conflict with each other. In Great Britain, the separate organization of hospital and community care, and health and social care, serves to compound these problems. The different approaches taken by these organizations, professions and academic disciplines have made it exceedingly difficult to address patients' needs in an integrated way. Health care education and delivery systems still suffer the unfortunate consequences of this, to the detriment of patient care.

Similar problems have beset psychology. Since the early twentieth century, psychological theory and research have developed into different schools of thought, each with their own theorists and researchers. Academic psychologists tend to focus on one discrete field of psychology with its own specialist network of communication via specialist journals and conferences. Thus a psychologist who specializes in one field of study, such as memory, may have little exposure to serious dialogue with those working in other areas of psychology. This makes it very difficult for those wishing to understand and apply psychological theory and research to their work in health or social care in an integrated way. It also means that many psychology textbooks can seem quite fragmented and confusing. In this chapter, we address the main schools of thought in psychology so that is possible to see where ideas in the psychology applied to health have come from. Each subsequent chapter addresses a different field of psychology with examples of how these can be applied to deliver effective health and social care.

The development of psychology

Before the twentieth century, the study of the mind was primarily the preserve of philosophers. This changed at the turn of the twentieth century with the emergence of psychology as a scientific discipline. As a natural science, psychology was dominated by positivist philosophy. According to **positivism**, human beings are objects of nature, sharing common functions or attributes that can be studied in an objective, scientific way.

Initially, the main methods of studying the mind were based on introspection and scientific experimentation. Introspection originated in philosophy and involves the analysis of one's own thoughts. Freud recognized the need for a more scientific approach and set about developing a more systematic method of studying the minds of others, which he termed **psychoanalysis**. Other researchers opted for laboratory-style experimentation to study behaviour change. This was termed behavioural psychology or **behaviourism**. Behaviourism involved the study of behaviour change under carefully controlled conditions. The 'subjects' of these experiments were predominantly rats and pigeons rather than humans, but it was assumed that the principles of learning observed in these experiments would apply equally to human beings. Another scientific approach to psychology was the study of human memory, which became part of cognitive psychology. Early experiments focused on the quantity of information that humans could remember under different conditions. Although based on human subjects, the experiments involved recalling nonsense syllables that were free of meaning.

In comparing these early approaches, it is evident that psychoanalysis captured the interest and imagination of those wanting to learn more about the nature of the human mind and its impact on human behaviour. Critics have since cast doubt on the scientific basis of psychoanalysis, but it has been very influential in a number of important areas, including the development of human relationships and coping with stress. Behaviourism and early memory research were criticized for the lack of real-world value (ecological validity), but many findings from these studies have informed the development of cognitive science and proved influential in health psychology. This is why they are included in this book

In the second half of the twentieth century, the scientific approach to psychology was appraised as problematic by Carl Rogers and fellow psychologists. Science is based on the assumption that people can be treated as objects of study and research findings generalized to the population under study. But Rogers claimed that each human is a unique individual who can only be understood in his or her own terms. He argued that it was inappropriate to regard people as objects of study, or to assume that an individual's response was predictable. Humanistic psychologists favoured an approach drawn from philosophy called 'existential phenomenology'. **Phenomenology** is not concerned with the development of universal laws or theories, but with understanding personal or subjective experience. It formed the basis of **humanistic psychology** which has proved very influential within the caring professions.

Another field of psychology to emerge during the twentieth century was social psychology. All other fields of psychology focused predominantly on individual thought and behaviour but largely ignored the social context in which people live and function. Social psychologists recognized the need to interpret behaviour in its social context. They set about conducting simulated and 'real-world' experiments that challenged many assumptions about how people think and behave in different types of social situation.

Towards the latter part of the twentieth century, psychoanalysis, behaviourism and humanistic psychology have become marginalized within academic psychology, though they are still influential in health and clinical psychology. The most prominent branch of academic psychology is now cognitive science. This is concerned with a scientific understanding of the human mind. It uses up-to-date technologies and links psychologists with those working in other disciplines such as artificial intelligence and neuroscience. One of the most influential aspects of cognitive science in the psychology of health is the development of a new discipline called **psychoneuroimmunology**. This seeks to understand the relationship between psychological factors and physiological responses that can affect health and illness (Chapter 7). Another new area of psychology of particular interest to the caring professions is narrative psychology, which focuses on both the content and coherence of autobiographical memories. You will find references to this in several chapters of this book.

Below, we explore the main schools of psychology in a little more detail.

Schools of thought in psychology

There are five main schools of thought in psychology in which academic psychologists normally work and on which health psychology is based. People working in the field of health or social care may draw on any or all of these, but it is helpful to understand the assumptions and principles that underpin them. They are:

- Cognitive science (also referred to as cognitive psychology): the study of **cognition** (mental processes) including memory, perception, information processing, psychophysiology and psychoneuroimmunology.
- Behavioural psychology (based on behaviourism): the study of learning by observing the direct effects of external environmental stimuli on behaviour and behaviour change.
- Psychodynamic psychology (developed from psychoanalysis): the study of the influence of childhood experiences on current psychological and emotional states.
- Humanistic psychology: the subjective study of human experience.
- Social psychology: the study of human behaviour in social settings.

Psychologists working in these different fields of psychology often agree that people tend to respond in predictable ways in certain clearly defined situations. What they usually disagree about is the theoretical explanation and interpretation of these observations.

Cognitive science

Cognitive psychology is concerned with thought processes. It was traditionally based on experimental studies of memory, perception and, more recently, information processing. Until the 1990s, cognitive theories were largely based on assumptions about how information might be transmitted and stored in the brain. More recently, the introduction of brain imaging techniques has enabled psychologists and neuroscientists to map this against brain function. As a result, cognitive psychology has been incorporated into cognitive science, which is now the dominant field of academic psychology.

Psychologists working in the field of psychoneuroimmunology are increasingly able to make direct links between psychosocial processes, immune function and health and illness (Chapter 7). In the field of mental health, cognitive-based therapies have emerged as important techniques to help change the way that psychologically distressed or behaviourally disturbed individuals interpret and respond to problem situations.

Unlike other schools of psychology, cognitive psychology or cognitive science is not associated with any one unifying theory or 'big name'. Instead, many psychologists are recognized for their special contributions to particular aspects of the discipline. However, in the field of treatment, Aaron Beck is best known for his theory of depression (Chapter 7) and the development of cognitive therapy as a treatment for depression.

Behavioural psychology

Behavioural psychology refers to the study of behavioural learning. It is based on the assumption that behaviour change is a direct response to changes in external stimuli and indicates that learning has taken place. Ivan Pavlov, working on research into animal digestion, was the first to report a simple form of associative learning which he termed **classical conditioning**. John Watson, often referred to as the father of behaviourism, went on to suggest that learning was the basic foundation of all human activity. Thus if it was possible to understand the process of learning, it would also be possible to develop universal laws to predict human behaviour. He proposed that psychologists should concentrate only on observable behaviour. They should not concern themselves with mental processes since (at that time) these could not be directly observed. Watson studied the effects of simple stimuli on reflex responses such as fear (Chapter 4). Behaviourism grew to greater prominence during the 1940s to 1970s with the work of B.F. Skinner on **operant conditioning**, which studied the effect of external stimuli on voluntary responses such as obtaining food. This led to the development of theories that predict a direct relationship between behaviour and its consequences.

During the 1980s, behavioural research became more sophisticated and enabled psychologists to draw inferences about the thought processes involved in behaviour change. Behavioural psychology declined in popularity for a number of reasons. Most of the research involved the use of animals, which became increasingly unacceptable to the general public. Researchers working in other areas of psychology questioned the applicability of animal experiments to human psychology, arguing that human mental processes are qualitatively different from those in other animal species. The assumption that human behaviour is determined by external forces (**determinism**) was challenged for philosophical and political reasons, since it seemed to contradict the notion of 'free will'. Finally, research in this field reached a point where it was possible to interpret learning in terms of underlying predictions or beliefs. As a result, important research in this field has been incorporated into cognitive science.

An important aspect of psychology to emerge from behavioural psychology was social learning theory, developed by Albert Bandura (Chapter 4). Bandura observed that certain aspects of human learning could not be accounted for by behaviourism. This included the ability to copy or model behavioural responses, based on observing how others behave in certain situations and what the consequences of their actions were. In other words, if Alex sees Jim getting praise from the teacher for getting a task right, then Alex is likely to copy Jim. Social learning theory focuses particularly on the learning of skills and has formed the basis of social cognition, on which much of health psychology is based.

Effective behaviour therapies have been developed for the treatment of fears and phobias, anxiety disorders and the management of unwanted or challenging behaviours (Chapter 4). **Cognitive behaviour therapy** has emerged as one of the most successful treatments of choice for non-psychotic disorders (those that do not involve disruption of rational thought processes). This incorporates behaviourist principles with those of cognitive therapy.

Psychodynamic psychology

Psychoanalysis was founded by Sigmund Freud as a 'scientific' way of understanding complex psychological problems. It was developed as a method of inquiry, a theory of mind and a mode of treatment. Freud was a medical doctor who studied neurological problems, later moving on to treat physical illnesses that were believed to be manifestations of psychological problems. The correct term for this is **psychogenic** illness (physical illness that has a psychological cause), as distinct from a **psychosomatic** disorder, which is a physical illness that has a psychological component (or vice versa).

The 'subjects' of Freud's investigations were people seeking therapeutic help for psychological or sometimes neurological problems. Central to his theory was the proposition that certain experiences during childhood are too uncomfortable to remember and are therefore 'repressed'. These repressed thoughts, which he proposed were commonly of a sexual nature, eventually give rise to a state of anxiety or depression which may be expressed in terms of physical symptoms. Freud believed that repressed thoughts are revealed through dreams, word associations, slips of the tongue and the interpretation of visual images. The exploration of repressed experiences, with the aid of the psychoanalyst, facilitates the release of repressed thoughts and feelings through processes such as trans-ference (expression of troublesome emotions directed at the therapist) and catharsis (release of negative emotions).

Psychoanalysis has had a tremendous influence on the ways in which people think and talk about motivations and unconscious processes. People commonly use Freudian terms and concepts, such as **denial** and **repression**, in everyday conversation, as though these are matters of fact rather than theoretical concepts. Similarly, the **ego** is also treated as something real. Freud's ideas have been influential in psychiatry, clinical psychology and counselling.

Without the benefit of modern medical technology, it is now clear that Freud was unable to diagnose some illnesses that were almost certainly genuine neurological diseases. Many aspects of psychoanalytic theory have not been amenable to experimental testing and have been difficult to prove or disprove. Psychoanalytic explanations are usually offered **post hoc** (after the event), and some would argue that psychoanalytic theory is there-fore unable to fulfil what they see as the prime purpose of a theory, to predict outcomes. This has led to attack from members of the scientific community who regard psychoanalysis as a **pseudoscience**.

Following Freud's death, psychoanalysis largely gave way to what was termed 'ego' psychology. This gave rise to a number of important developmental and cognitive theories, including Erikson's theory of life stage development (Chapter 2), theories of attachment, separation and loss (Chapter 5) and coping theory (Chapter 7). It also led to the development of **psychodynamic** psychotherapy.

Psychodynamic psychotherapy evolved from psychoanalysis under the influence of Melanie Klein and others. It emphasizes processes of development and change and retains the proposition that most emotional problems are caused by unresolved difficulties in relationships encountered in childhood. However, most psychodynamic therapists reject the notion of the sexual urge as the prime cause of repressed thoughts. They base their therapy on helping clients to retrieve and resolve difficult or traumatic memories, many of which are related to difficulties in the caregiver–child attachment relationship. However, this approach to therapy has given rise to some concerns about the possibility of introducing false memories.

Psychodynamic counselling is currently one of the most popular approaches in western societies to the treatment of anxiety and depression. Psychodynamic psychology has also been influential in the development of a number of important theories in other areas of psychology. These include attachment theory in developmental psychology, and certain theories of coping with stress. Unlike some other aspects of psychodynamic or psychoanalytic theory, these are amenable to scientific testing.

Humanistic psychology

Humanistic psychology has its origins in existential **phenomenology** in which causal explanations are of relatively little interest. Humanistic psychologists do not deny the existence of an objective external reality, but are concerned with individual perceptions and interpretations which are influenced by social and cultural meanings and past experiences. They acknowledge that individual perceptions may change over time and vary in different social and cultural settings. Psychologists who accept this philosophical view reject the scientific method as an appropriate method of investigation. They would argue that there is no single truth, no single 'right' way of doing things, and no 'one size fits all' treatment for emotional problems.

The main focus of humanistic psychology is on the individual's sense of self (Chapter 2). Carl Rogers is most commonly associated with this aspect of humanistic psychology. He trained as a psychoanalyst and worked with people who had emotional problems, but eventually rejected psychoanalysis. He noted that people who came to him with psychological problems exhibited a natural tendency towards growth and maturity that enabled them to overcome many of their own problems. Therefore, he encouraged people to explore their self-understanding. Rogers introduced the concept of **self-actualization** which he used to refer to an innate tendency that drives all individuals to achieve their full potential within the limits of environmental or situational constraints.

An important theoretical contribution to humanistic psychology came from Abraham Maslow in the 1950s. Maslow observed human needs in different settings and used these to construct a 'hierarchy of needs' (see Figure 1.1). He predicted that for all people, lower-order needs (such as basic needs for food, drink and warmth), must be satisfied before higher-order (intellectual) needs can be fulfilled. Unlike Rogers, who conceptualized self-actualization as a process, Maslow described it as the pinnacle of human achievement. Self-actualization includes accepting self and others for what they are; the ability to tolerate uncertainty; creativity; the use of problem-centred rather than self-centred approaches to dealing with issues; and strong moral and ethical standards. Yet it is actually very difficult to identify if or when someone has attained that state. Maslow's hierarchy has provided the theoretical basis for much work in the human professions, including nursing, education and management, and forms the basis of many models of nursing. However, it is not popular with academic psychologists because it lacks scientific evidence.

Rogers used his clinical observations to develop Rogerian counselling, which is a client-centred therapy. He recognized that, given freedom and opportunity, people often spontaneously reveal their own concerns and usually have sufficient insight to identify the solutions to their own problems. The task of the therapist is to enable or facilitate this process. Rogerian counsellors act in a non-judgemental, non-directive way, displaying warmth, empathy and 'unconditional personal regard' for their clients. Humanistic counselling is quite different from psychodynamic counselling in that the therapist makes no attempt to interpret the client's problems or direct a course of action.

At the beginning of the twenty-first century, Rogerian counselling appears to have lost ground in popularity to psychodynamic counselling. Nevertheless, humanistic principles remain central to the notion of the **therapeutic relationship**, which is built on the notion of accepting people for what or who they are in a non-judgemental way.

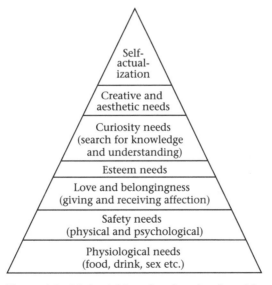

Figure 1.1 Maslow's hierarchy of needs, adapted from Maslow (1970).

Social psychology

Much of social psychology lies in a grey area between psychology, sociology and anthropology. Social psychologists seek to explain how humans behave in certain social contexts and predict social influences on human thought and behaviour. Research in social psychology includes games and experiments that manipulate 'real-world' type situations to see how people respond. This often involves some degree of deception because people tend to change their behaviour if they think they are being observed. We describe some of these experiments in Chapters 2 and 6 because they have important implications for people working in health care settings. Social psychologists also use participant observation to study people's responses in naturalistic settings. In the field of health and social care, social psychology has done much to enhance our understanding of the interactions between health professionals and patients. It has also contributed much to our understanding of the ways in which individuals make sense of illness and disability, and how those with altered minds or bodies are perceived by others.

Psychological facts versus psychological theory

In spite of recent advances in brain technology, it is rarely possible to study the human mind directly. We can never 'know' what someone is really thinking. We can only find out by studying what people say, how people behave and, more recently, how the electrical activity in their brains varies in different situations. Therefore, psychology, as with all social sciences, is not a body of 'facts', but a body of theories that changes over time in the light of new information, new research methods, new technologies and new ways of thinking about things.

What is a theory?

The purpose of scientific theory is not merely to explain what has happened in the past, but to predict and control what will happen in the future. For example, while it is helpful to be able to explain why people get ill, the main use of health-related theory should be to prevent them from becoming ill in the first place. Similarly, the main purpose of psychology is to be able to predict and control certain aspects of human beliefs and behaviour.

The test of a good scientific theory, according to Karl Popper, a famous twentieth-century philosopher of science, is that it must be clear and concise (this is known as the principle of parsimony, or 'Occam's razor'). A good theory should also be falsifiable. Popper argued that no theory can ever be proved, but it can be disproved. He used the example of white swans. It is possible to observe thousands of swans over many years and record that they are all white. The logical deduction is that all swans are white. But it takes only one black swan to completely destroy the theory that all swans are white. A theory generates a logical statement or **hypothesis** that may be supported by evidence but, according to Popper, can never be proved. Therefore, a theory is not a fact.

Psychological theory, as with all scientific theory, must be treated with caution. Theories predict only what is likely to happen. Quantitative research tests predictions at the level of statistical probability. This tells us only what is likely to occur in the population that has been studied, not what will happen to a single individual. People vary in their responses, so no theory or research evidence can ever tell us precisely what will apply to an individual person or patient. Therefore, when applying theory to practice, it is always necessary to apply IF–THEN logic. For example 'If this theory is correct, then the following course of action is likely to be appropriate . . .' or 'If X theory is applied, then this patient may be at risk of . . .'.

Research methods in psychology

Research methods are the ways by which theories are tested and new knowledge gained. The main methods used in psychology are given below.

Quantitative methods

Quantitative methods are usually designed to test a hypothesis or prediction, based on a theory. For example, a theory might predict that a particular set of beliefs will produce a certain type of behaviour; or a particular psychological intervention will lead to a certain outcome. These methods are termed **deductive** (or hypothetico-deductive). Quantitative methods require that psychological outcomes are measurable (see also Chapter 8).

The development of psychological outcome measures

Instruments are constructed to measure each psychological concept, such as anxiety or self-efficacy. These instruments consist of a series of statements or questions (items) that each represent different aspects of the concept. A fixed range of responses to each item are offered, as in a **Likert scale** or **semantic differential** scale. Once tested for their **validity** and **reliability**, these instruments are used to measure outcomes in experiments and to test the relationship between a range of variables or factors in questionnaire or interview surveys (see Bowling 1997).

Experimental methods

The scientific method most commonly used to test theory is the experiment. An experiment involves the measurement of a set of responses to an intervention. A health care intervention consists of the manipulation of a condition, such as the introduction of a new treatment, or a change in circumstance or environment. The experimental design advocated in the biomedical sciences to test health care interventions is the randomized controlled trial (RCT). Ideally, neither the researcher nor the patient should know which treatment option (active or control) the patient is receiving. This is called 'blinding'. Blinding is used to ensure that patients' expectations do not lead to a **placebo response** that favours a particular intervention. But in testing psychosocial interventions, it is impossible for the therapist or client not to be aware which treatment is used. Outcomes may be biased in favour of the intervention unless the control group receive an alternative treatment that is perceived as entirely comparable, which is difficult.

Social psychologists often use naturalistic or field experiments to develop theories about how people respond in different situations. A naturalistic experiment is one that is located in a 'real-life' type of situation but where, unknown to participants, the researcher manipulates what actually happens. The results help to identify what it is about a situation that affects beliefs, attitudes and behaviour.

Survey methods

Survey methods use structured interviews or questionnaires as instruments to collect self-report data about such issues as health-related beliefs and behaviours. This allows the researcher to identify patterns of response within a population, differences in response between groups (for example, men and women), and relationships between variables, such as the relationship between beliefs and behaviours. The method is very popular in health psychology. For example, it is possible to test the relationship between the belief that 'exercise is important for health' and the age of the respondent. The findings might then be used to identify different approaches to intervention for different age groups. Although surveys are used to test psychological theory, it is impossible to distinguish cause from effect when the data are cross-sectional (collected from a population at a single point in time). Longitudinal methods in which data are collected from the same people at different points in time make it possible to distinguish cause from effect.

Observation methods

Social psychologists and anthropologists use observation methods to construct theories about how people behave in different situations. For example, a good way to study the behaviour of patients in out-patient departments is to go and sit in the department and record what goes on. It is possible to measure such things as the effect of different seating arrangements, or to record the frequency and nature of interpersonal interactions.

Observation methods may be qualitative (recording the type of interactions and nature of responses) as well as quantitative.

Qualitative methods

Qualitative methods usually seek to describe or explain phenomena, and may be used to generate new theory. They are therefore termed **inductive** methods. It is difficult to produce explanations that are not based on preconceived thoughts or ideas. Therefore the researcher must be aware of this and try to approach data collection and analysis with an open mind. Data collection may involve semi-structured or unstructured interviews, observations or documentary analysis. The data presented in qualitative research reports are usually in the form of direct quotations or rich description, rather than statistics, and are often easier to read and understand. They often challenge existing assumptions and make a real contribution to our understanding of patients' needs, and the nature of patient and staff interactions. There are a range of different qualitative methods that are used to explore different types of issues.

Phenomenology led to the development of phenomenological research methods. These use qualitative interviews to understand the 'lived experience' of various aspects of life, including health and illness, without imposing any preconceived ideas. It involves, for example, listening to patients' accounts of their illnesses without imposing questions that restrict or direct their line of thought. Within health psychology, interpretive phenomenology has become a popular qualitative method for understanding the patient experience of disease or illness. Discourse analysis is a popular research method for understanding the influence of language on dialogue. Narrative analysis is used to investigate the structure as well as the content of people's stories about events in their lives. These methods have supported the emergence of two new areas of study called 'discursive psychology' and 'narrative psychology'. Psychologists also use qualitative methods drawn from other disciplines. For example, grounded theory was developed by sociologists and uses data from a variety of interview, observation and documented sources to construct new theoretical accounts of social phenomena. Ethnography is derived from anthropology and is concerned with understanding and comparing different cultural groups using observation methods.

Pop psychology and pseudoscience

It is important to discriminate between psychology as a serious academic discipline and 'pop psychology'. It is often said that psychology is just common sense. But there are many examples where common sense is contradicted by good psychological research. Much of what we think of as psychology has no scientific foundation and is therefore myth. An example is the commonly held belief that when patients complain about a symptom for which there is no confirmable medical diagnosis, it must be 'all in the mind'.

This assumption is unsafe unless or until a detailed assessment of the individual and their situation has been conducted.

A pseudoscience is one that has a body of knowledge or theory that cannot be tested or has never been tested. For example, some psychologists tend to regard psychoanalysis as a pseudoscience because it has generated some complex theory that has been difficult to test. In an age of 'evidence-based health care' it is important to be careful about applying any aspect of psychology unless there is reasonable evidence to support it.

Psychology in practice: Introduction to scenario

In order to understand psychology, it is important to appreciate how it can be applied in different contexts. Therefore we have devised a family scenario that will be used throughout the book to provide examples, as in a soap opera. Figure 1.2 contains a family tree for the 'psychosoap' family. We have also included a thumbnail sketch of each family member to help you make sense of the examples.

Anna is currently on a diploma programme at university, training to be a nurse.

Anna has a brother, Jo (short for Jonah), who has drifted since leaving school at the age of 16. He is currently unemployed and living with his girlfriend, Sasha, and her son, Lee. Sasha is pregnant with Jo's baby.

Janice and Mark are parents to Anna and Jo. Mark recently retired early from his job as a groundsman because of the onset of type 2 diabetes, hypertension and angina. Janice works as a health care assistant in a local nursing home.

Janice's mother, Margaret, was divorced 25 years ago and lives on her own in a town not far from Janice and Mark. She was born in the West Indies and came to the United Kingdom in the 1950s, where she married Fred who was then a postman. They separated nearly 30 years ago and he died in 1989.

Mark's father, Ted, is a former factory worker. He is a widower whose wife died 3 years ago. He has chronic heart disease and has recently given up his home to live with Janice and Mark.

Mark's sister Lillian is unmarried and lives alone close by. She has been unwell and has recently been undergoing medical tests.

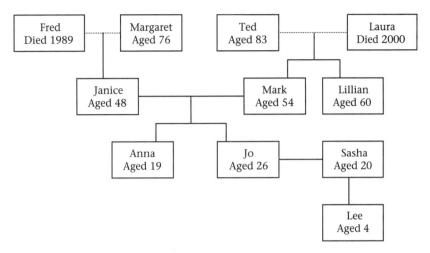

Figure 1.2 'Psychosoap' family tree.

Applying psychology to explain Anna's anxiety

In order to assist in understanding the implications of different schools of thought in psychology, we have applied each in turn to try to make sense of a common situation in which Anna is the central character. Consider the following:

> Anna has just joined the university as a student nurse and has to give her first seminar presentation to her tutor group. Although other students have all seemed a bit nervous, they have all delivered their seminars without too much fuss. Anna delayed her presentation because she was anxious about doing it. As her turn approaches, she is increasingly panic-stricken. It gets so bad that it could threaten Anna's future career. How can Anna's anxiety be understood, and what approaches are available to help her to overcome it?

Anxiety includes physiological responses caused by the arousal of the autonomic nervous system. These include an increase in pulse and blood pressure, sweating, and the impulse to urinate or defecate. Anna's physiological responses indicate that she is very anxious.

Cognitive approaches to Anna's anxiety

In attempting to explain Anna's anxiety, a cognitive scientist might be interested in making sense of Anna's problem-solving processes. How does she interpret the demands of the task and her ability to perform it?

Cognitive approaches focus on the interpretation of the task and planning an appropriate strategy to deal with it. Anna is quite capable of doing what all of her classmates have done. She may have underestimated her ability to create and present a seminar or has set herself a very high standard. A cognitive therapist would wish to help Anna change her beliefs about the demands of the task and her ability to perform it successfully. The therapist would work with Anna to encourage her to be realistic about the standard of work expected at this level and to think positively about her own ability to perform the task successfully. Anna may lack the problem-solving skills to produce the seminar successfully, in which case the therapist would encourage Anna to set about the task in a more structured way. This might include something as simple as writing out a summary of the content on a series of prompt cards.

Behavioural and social learning approaches to Anna's anxiety

Behaviourists might explain Anna's anxiety in terms of the outcomes of past experiences in similar situations. For example, she may have felt humiliated when she was unable to answer a question correctly in class at school. However, rather than dwell on these beliefs, a behaviour therapist would focus on providing positive feedback on actions related to the task. The therapist might encourage the learning of relaxation skills to counteract feelings of anxiety and then provide Anna with opportunities to rehearse her seminar in a safe environment, while practising relaxation. This aims to increase her confidence in her ability to undertake the task successfully (this is termed **self-efficacy**). First, she might watch others perform the task. Then she would rehearse it on her own, then in comfortable surroundings with the therapist or a close friend, then in an empty classroom with the same therapist or friend and then with a few friends. This would gradually increase her confidence and reduce her anxiety so that when she finally has to present the seminar to her tutor group she feels relaxed and confident.

Psychodynamic approaches to Anna's anxiety

A psychodynamic therapist would be interested to find out why Anna is so anxious. In exploring her childhood experiences, they might find, for example, that Anna's father had been very strict and critical and had set very high standards which she found difficult to live up to. Her mother had always wanted Anna to train as a nurse, since she herself had not had that opportunity. As a result, Anna finds herself under a lot of pressure to succeed. She is frightened of giving the seminar because she fears that it will not be up the standard she expects of herself and feels afraid of letting down the family. The psychodynamic therapist might seek to explore the origins of these feelings with her and, in so doing, seek to release her from her feelings of anxiety.

Humanistic approaches to Anna's anxiety

A humanistic counsellor would seek to help Anna explore the reasons for her anxiety in her own terms, and to help her resolve it in her own way. They would make no prior assumptions about the causes of the problem. Rather they would encourage Anna to talk about her anxiety and her thoughts about seminar presentation. If she sees herself as less competent than others at giving seminar presentations, they would encourage her to explore why this is and might encourage her to role-play someone who is more confident. Having demonstrated that she is quite capable of accomplishing the seminar presentation in her new confident persona, her sense of self-worth and confidence are likely to improve, enabling her to give the seminar. This will enhance her personal development and her journey towards self-actualization.

Social psychological approaches to Anna's anxiety

A social psychologist might identify that Anna makes negative comparisons between herself and the other students, seeing herself not just as less able, but as less presentable. Giving a seminar is not just about content but about personal presentation, and much anxiety is generated because we are afraid of what other people will think of us. In this case, the social psychologist might suggest that she uses new props to help her feel more confident and attract social approval: for example, having her hair done, dressing and making up carefully, and preparing material that will entertain her audience.

Comparing different psychological approaches to Anna's anxiety

It can be seen from these brief analyses that these psychological approaches are very different in their explanations and interpretations of the same phenomenona. It cannot be said that one is right and one is wrong. But it may be that different approaches are appropriate for different people, depending on the problems they have and the ways they prefer to deal with them. Many psychologists working in the fields of therapy or counselling use what is termed an **eclectic** approach. This means that they assess the nature and extent of the problem and then use whichever tools are most appropriate to assist the individual and overcome the problem. Equally, those in need of help are likely to select a therapist with whom they feel able to develop a rapport and an approach that best suits their personal preferences.

One treatment not considered above, but which might be the treatment of choice had Anna consulted her doctor, is the use of antidepressant medication. This might be unlikely for anxiety limited to seminar presentation, but would probably be considered if Anna had reported to her doctor that she was unable to cope at university and was feeling anxious and depressed. Drug treatments for anxiety and depression are based upon a medical model that conceptualizes anxiety and depression as illnesses.

Antidepressants alter brain chemistry and make people feel less anxious and depressed. In so doing, the individual is able to tackle problems that they previously felt unable to address. However, drugs do not necessarily solve problems or enhance skills and it is important that, where necessary, consideration is given to supportive therapeutic interventions such as those mentioned above. This ensures that there is no relapse once the individual stops taking the tablets. Sources of help available for Anna and others with actual or potential psychological problems are described below.

Professionals involved in the prevention, management and treatment of psychological problems

The number of psychologists working in health and social care and other fields has increased considerably over the last few decades. Their tasks focus on preventing, assessing, treating and/or helping individuals to manage emotional, behavioural and cognitive problems using psychological theory and research. They also work alongside, or provide consultancy to, other health professionals. It is helpful to be able to distinguish between the skills available to different types of therapists who use psychology. Definitions of psychologists given below are taken from the website of the British Psychological Society, www.bps.org.uk/, from where further details can be obtained.

Clinical psychologist: aims to reduce psychological distress and enhance and promote psychological well-being. They work with people with mental or physical health problems, which might include anxiety and depression, serious and enduring mental illness, adjustment to physical illness, neurological disorders, addictive behaviours, childhood behaviour disorders, personal and family relationships. They work with people throughout the lifespan, including with those with severe learning difficulties.

Health psychologist: applies psychological research and methods to the prevention and management of disease, the promotion and maintenance of health, the identification of psychological factors that contribute to physical illness, and the formulation of health policy. As examples, they study why and when people seek professional advice about their health, why they do or do not take preventative measures, how patients and health care professionals interact, how patients adapt to illness, and the links between perception, health behaviour and physical functioning.

Counselling psychologist: applies psychology to working collaboratively with people across a diverse range of human problems. This includes helping people manage difficult life events such as bereavement, past and present relationships, and working with mental health issues and disorders. Counselling psychologists accept subjective experience as valid for each person, explore underlying issues and use an active collaborative relationship to empower people to consider change.

Counselling psychologists utilize a holistic stance, which involves examining issues within the wider context of what has given rise to them.

The roles of psychologists overlap with the roles of other health care professionals who have similar aims, including:

Counsellor: Similar to a counselling psychologist, except that anyone can describe themselves as a counsellor. Training courses vary from a few days to several years. There are short courses that provide a certificate of attendance, longer courses that provide a 'certificate' or 'diploma' (though the academic level may be unspecified), and MSc programmes that include a period of supervised training. Some training programmes offer an eclectic mix of psychological approaches, though most follow a particular psychological model such as Rogerian or psychodynamic counselling.

Psychoanalyst: Someone who has trained in psychoanalysis under the supervision of an approved psychoanalyst. All approved psychoanalysts can trace the provenance of their trainers back to those who were trained directly by Freud himself. All analysts undergo psychoanalysis themselves as part of a lengthy period of training.

Psychodynamic psychotherapist: A therapist who has undergone a period of intensive training, including personal analysis and supervised practice, and who bases their approach on a **psychodynamic** model.

Psychiatrist: a medical doctor who, since qualifying, has specialized in the diagnosis and treatment of people with mental health disorders. They may use a range of psychological therapies, but these usually include drug treatment which they have the right to prescribe. They sometimes use physical interventions such as ECT (electroconvulsive therapy). They are in charge of psychiatric beds and have the authority to admit people to hospital for treatment. They usually assume the clinical lead of a multiprofessional mental health team that normally includes clinical psychologists, mental health nurses and social workers.

Cognitive behavioural therapist: a qualified health care professional, such as a mental health nurse, who has completed undergraduate or postgraduate specialist training in **cognitive behavioural therapy** (CBT) for the treatment for such disorders as depression, psychosis or obsessive-compulsive disorders. All clinical psychologists are trained to offer CBT.

Summary of key points

- Psychology is the study of human behaviour, thought processes and emotions.
- The study of psychology is important to help us understand ourselves, the people we work with and the people we care for.
- We have discussed five main approaches to psychology: behaviourism;

cognitive psychology; psychodynamic theories; humanistic psychology; and social psychology.

- Different approaches to psychology may be based on different sets of assumptions about the nature of human beings, have different ways of explaining human thought and behaviour, use different methods of research and offer different approaches to therapy.
- Each approach to psychology offers a unique contribution to our understanding of health, illness and human interaction in health care.
- Psychology is used by a range of psychologists and other professionals working in fields related to mental and physical health care, social care, and health promotion.
- A scenario is used as an aid to understanding and application of psychology.

Further reading

Background information about the nature of psychology and the schools of thought in psychology is to be found in any introductory undergraduate textbook on psychology. It is strongly recommended that a recent edition be used, for example:

Gross, R. (2001) *Psychology: The Science of Mind and Behaviour*, 4th edition. London: Hodder and Stoughton.

THE PERCEPTION OF SELF AND OTHERS

- What is the 'self'?
- How do we learn about and understand our 'self'?
- What are the social influences on the way we behave and present ourselves?
- What do we mean by 'attitudes'?
- What influences stigmatization and prejudice?
- Why do we justify our own behaviour differently from the way we explain other people's behaviour?
- Do personality traits provide a useful way of categorizing people?

Introduction

In this chapter, we explore perhaps one of the most interesting concepts in psychology, the sense of 'self'. This is particularly important in health and social care because we are often dealing with people whose sense of self and self-worth has been changed or damaged in some way by illness, disease or disability. Further, in the context of health and social care, we need to be aware of the ways in which other people perceive us and what influences their impressions of us. We start by considering what self means and how we come to acquire our sense of who we are.

The self concept

It seems to be part of human nature to wonder exactly who or what we are. There are so many ways to describe ourselves: what we look like, how we feel in different types of situation, how we behave towards others, what we do at work, what roles we have in the family or society. At the beginning of the twenty-first century, people seem to be obsessed with the need to feel good about themselves, to the extent that well-known figures have spent years 'in therapy' or sought to change their bodies through cosmetic surgery. Present-day western societies place great emphasis on the body: its size, shape, complexion, hairstyle and adornments including clothing, jewellery, piercings and tattoos. But what do these really tell us about ourselves and others? How do we gain our sense of self?

Psychological theories are dominated by western cultural beliefs that view the 'self' as a discrete and personal entity. In western cultures, the worth of an individual is commonly defined in terms of having a good job, earning a lot of money, and owning a nice house or smart car. In contrast, other cultures emphasize the collective nature of human beings and their embeddedness in social systems. Individual worth in such cultures has traditionally been judged by the individual's contribution to family and community. In this chapter, we focus on psychological theories that explain how we come to understand ourselves and then review some of the social influences on our perceptions of ourselves and others.

The looking-glass self

We all have our own theories about ourselves and probably most of us assume that our self-understanding is gained through a process of **introspection** or personal reflection. But an early explanation of the development of the self concept, and one that is still widely respected, was offered by Cooley in 1902. He proposed the notion of 'the looking-glass self'. According to Cooley, the concept of self develops through social interaction. He argued that our sense of personal identity is a reflection of how we are regarded and responded to by other people. For example, other people confer labels on us, such as good-looking or hard-working. We internalize these labels and use them to define ourselves in relation to others. Positive labels make us feel good about ourselves and can motivate us to do well. Negative labels make us feel bad about ourselves and can reduce our belief in ourselves.

Most of us can remember some of the labels placed on us by our parents and others during childhood. These are often used to distinguish between siblings. In the scenario family (Chapter 1), Anna was labelled the one who worked hard, while her younger brother Jo was labelled lazy. Such labels may or may not reflect the 'truth', but can become self-fulfilling prophecies. This may help to explain why Anna is anxious to work hard and achieve success in her training as a nurse, while Jo failed to achieve at school and is currently unemployed. This type of explanation suggests that what is commonly referred to as 'personality' is not just a consequence of inherited disposition but is substantially created or modified by our interaction with those around us. You may care to reflect on the labels placed on you as you were growing up and consider the impact these might have had on your life.

Self defined by social comparison

Leon Festinger (1954), a social psychologist, introduced social comparison theory which proposes that we construct our sense of self by making comparisons with important others. For example, that someone is 5 feet 8 inches tall is a statement of fact. But whether they consider themselves tall or short depends on whom they compare themselves with. They might consider themselves tall if a women and short if a man; short if American and tall if Japanese (though these stereotypes are now somewhat outdated). Downward social comparisons (seeing oneself as better than others) tends to boost self-esteem (feeling of self-worth) and maintain a sense of well-being. For example, people who are older or disabled are often heard to comment that there are others who are worse off. This seems to help them to feel better about their own situation.

When we are young, we tend to accept the labels others confer upon us. But as we get older, we make our own comparisons with those who are important to us. Much of our self concept and self-esteem depends on the choice of an appropriate **reference group**. Thus someone who gains a place at the University of Poppleton might consider themselves very successful if they are from a family with no history of going to university, but a failure if they are from a family where there is a strong tradition of winning Oxbridge scholarships.

According to social identity theory (Tajfel 1982), one's identity results from a balance between a need to be similar to one's reference group and the need to be a unique individual. This means that we can have more than one identity, for example, a personal identity and a group identity. Children are very aware of the need for a group identity and are often afraid of dressing or acting differently from their peers. As they approach their teens, they often seem torn between the need to assert their own individual identity and the need to conform to their reference group. Therefore, distinctive group identities seem to emerge at this time. These identities are associated with particular styles of dressing and behaving.

Anna in the family scenario has recently acquired a new identity as a nurse. With this comes a uniform, bedside manner, code of conduct, and set of public expectations. But when she goes off duty and out with her friends, she will assume a quite different identity. The identities we confer on others, based on our assumptions about them, are often rejected by them. For example, if you talk to older people, you will often find that many reject the notion that they are old and will tend to distance themselves from other older people. A 90-year-old might refer to an 80-year-old as 'that poor old soul'. Many older people decline to join seniors clubs because they just do not identify with 'them'. It becomes clear that, in many circumstances, people just do not see themselves the same way that others see them. Therefore it is inappropriate to refer to 'these people', as though people share common characteristics according to a particular group membership.

George Kelly's personal construct theory

George Kelly was a psychologist and psychotherapist commonly associated with humanistic psychology. Kelly (1955) proposed that, as we grow up, we learn about ourselves and the world around us in much the same way as scientists produce and test theories. According to Kelly, we organize this knowledge into a series of dimensions which he called 'constructs'. These constructs define our sense of self. Each represents a continuum between a positive and negative pole. For example, Anna might choose to describe herself as rather dull, as opposed to interesting; quite plain, rather than attractive; and very shy, rather than outgoing.

Kelly developed the 'repertory grid' technique as a method of assessing an individual's personal constructs or sense of self. He proposed that many psychological problems are a consequence of discrepancies between our concept of an ideal self and our perceptions of our actual self. An example of a repertory grid applied to Anna is given in Figure 2.1.

	Myself as I am (actual self)	Myself as I would like to be (ideal self)	Brother	Best friend
Interesting (✓) Dull (✗)	✗	✓	✓	✓
Attractive (✓) Plain (✗)	✗	✓	✓	✓
Outgoing (✓) Shy (✗)	✗	✓	✓	✓

Figure 2.1   Anna's repertory grid.

Anna selected the three key constructs to describe herself and two people to compare herself with. In the example, Anna rates herself less positively than others on all three dimensions. If this led her to feel depressed, a therapist might work with her to focus on her positive characteristics, and encourage her to try out new roles that facilitate positive comparisons with others.

Kelly emphasized that people's views of reality are important in guiding their behaviour. Sometimes, false comparisons are associated with serious health consequences.

Anna's friend, Clare, suffers from anorexia. She judges herself to be fat in relation to her ideal self when she is in fact very underweight in relation to population norms. This leads her to continue to diet in order to lose even more weight.

Personal construct theory is now less commonly used in academic or therapeutic settings. But the principles are useful in helping people to understand how distorted beliefs about the self can contribute to mental health problems.

Self and narrative

A recent development in psychology has been what is termed **narrative psychology**, which is based on personal accounts or stories. One of the earliest proponents of listening to patients' stories as a way of finding out about adjustment to illness was Arthur Kleinman, a psychiatrist and anthropologist. His classic book, *The Illness Narratives* (Kleinman 1988) focused on what it is like to live with chronic pain. The importance of narrative has been recognized in sociology (Frank 1995) and gerontology (Kenyon and Randall 2001). These authors argue that we are the stories we tell. We each have our own unique life story that encompasses the past, present and future. These represent our map and our destination or purpose. Our narrative defines us as someone who is unique and distinguishes us from others. Our story may not be entirely factual because, as Murray (2003) explains, we construct a narrative to make sense of our life experiences. Narrative provides a sense of continuity over time. We use it to justify our actions and our existence.

Major life-changing events, including chronic illness, disability or loss, cause biographical disruption and challenge the existing sense of self (Radley 1994; see also Chapter 5). In the face of such events, we may have to change our narrative or 'restory' our lives to accommodate a different and unforeseen outcome. Thus it is possible that life changes can lead to a new or changed sense of self. Frank argued that a story demands a listener; therefore the narrative self is one to be heard, rather than measured. Allowing (but not forcing) people to tell their stories or review their lives is emerging as an important approach to therapy for those who have experienced life-changing events or situations (Chapters 5 and 7). Constructing a meaningful narrative may help to improve sense of self-worth and facilitate what Antonovsky (1985) termed a sense of coherence, which is amenable to measurement (Chapter 7).

Narrative therapy

Narrative writing has been shown to be an effective alternative to counselling. James Pennebaker (1993) developed a very simple intervention that has been shown to be associated with significant improvements in health and well-being. These are the instructions:

> For the next four days, I would like you to spend about twenty minutes each day writing about your very deepest thoughts and feelings about the most traumatic experience of your life. In your writing, I'd like you to really let go and explore your very deepest emotion and thoughts. You might link your topic to your relationships with others, to your past, your present or your future, or to how you have been, who you would like to be or who you are now. You may write about the same general issues each day, or about something different. All of your writing will be completely confidential.

The outcomes of this simple intervention appear impressive. It has been tested with university students, Holocaust survivors, prisoners, crime victims, arthritis and chronic pain sufferers, the unemployed and those with post-traumatic stress disorder. The results show significant improvements in psychological well-being, coping, immune function, physical health and reduced visits to medical services (Pennebaker and Seagal 1999; Esterling *et al.* 1999). Various explanations for its effectiveness have been proposed. Writing may help individuals to set traumatic events in context and regain a **sense of coherence** (see Chapters 5 and 7).

Self-esteem

Self-esteem reflects a critical personal evaluation of self-worth and is a central component of psychological well-being. Theories of self-esteem depend very much on the field of psychology they are drawn from. For example, according to personal construct theory, self-esteem reflects the degree of discrepancy between the ideal and actual self (little discrepancy is associated with high self-esteem). A psychodynamic psychologist may view self-esteem as resulting from attachment relationships formed in early life. According to social learning theory, self-esteem reflects the extent to which an individual feels their actions influence the world around them and enable them to achieve their aims in life. These explanations are different but not mutually exclusive.

Drawing on social comparison and social identity theory, self-esteem is influenced by how we believe others view us, together with how much we value their judgements. This is termed the **social norm**. If we value the judgements of important others, we are more likely to take notice of their attitudes towards us (see Chapter 8 on health-related behaviours). People with low self-esteem often lack confidence even when they are much admired by those around them. This may be because they do not recognize themselves as having desired attributes. Feedback on self-worth commences at birth and is particularly important during the formative years. Therefore childhood experiences in the family and in peer groups are very important in determining self-esteem. Changes in adult life, including loss of job or job promotion, forming a new relationship or marital breakdown, gaining a new skill or loss of ability, or injuries or alterations to the body or body image, can all have positive or negative effects on self-esteem. The current trend towards cosmetic surgery illustrates the effect of positive body image on self-esteem. Equally, changes brought about by disease or injury can damage self-esteem.

Self-esteem may also be influenced by the roles that are important to the individual. For example, a mastectomy scar may damage self-esteem in the role of lover, but be of little importance in the role of, say, an accountant. Of course, people's roles change throughout their lives, and this raises questions about whether self-esteem is stable throughout life or whether it changes. Research evidence supports the view that there are stable elements to self-esteem which are formed early in life, but that life experiences may serve to raise or lower self-esteem (Rubin and Hewstone 1998). An example of the type of change that can affect self-esteem is alteration to body image.

Al-Ghazal *et al.* (2000) compared the impact of different types of breast surgery (local excision, mastectomy and mastectomy plus breast reconstruction) on measures that included body image and self-esteem for women aged between 20 and 70. Perhaps not surprisingly, they found that cosmetic outcome was closely associated with psychological outcome. In all age groups, mastectomy was associated with poorer body image and lower self-esteem. As a result of this and previous findings, the team of researchers concluded that breast reconstruction should automatically be offered to all women undergoing mastectomy. However, this was a retrospective study and the findings may have been influenced by treatment preference. An earlier prospective study by Morris and Ingham (1988) indicated that providing choice, rather than the type of operation performed, led to improved physical and psychological functioning.

According to Bandura's social learning theory (Bandura 1997), self-esteem comes from the confidence in one's ability to achieve important goals. This is usually the result of one's own endeavours, but may also be a consequence of collective effort. However, Abrams and Hogg (2004) caution that individualism versus collectivism is culturally influenced. Therefore self-efficacy may only be an important determinant of self-esteem in western societies that value individual effort and personal achievement. Overall, it appears that self-esteem is strongly influenced by the perceived ability to meet both personal and social group expectations. Those who set a high level of personal expectation or experience negative social feedback, particularly during childhood, are more likely to develop low self-esteem. One reason why adolescents form groups or gangs may be to boost their collective sense of self-esteem by setting their own rules for achievement.

Body image

Our bodies are important determinants of our self concept. Bodies have certain unique features that remain relatively stable over time and by which other people recognize us. Other body features change with age and life experiences. As health professionals, we work with many people who have to deal not just with important life changes but with changes to their actual bodies. Some of these are abrupt changes resulting from trauma, disease processes or surgery. Other changes are insidious, as in disease processes such as rheumatoid arthritis or chronic heart disease. Both types of change to the body can result in the need to change the self concept and may seriously challenge an individual's sense of identity.

According to Price (1990) normal body image has three parts: body reality, body ideal and body presentation. Body reality refers to the physical structure of the individual body, whether an individual is tall or short, fat or slim, fair or dark, etc. The structure of the body changes over time, from infancy to childhood, through sexual differentiation at puberty, through middle age (and the menopause for women), into old age. At different periods in our lives, we appear to inhabit very different bodies although, paradoxically, most people have a sense of continuity about their own bodies. Basic aspects of our body reality are determined by genetic factors such as eye and hair colour, height and body shape. But body reality can be changed deliberately, for example, by going on a slimming diet or having cosmetic surgery. It may also be changed as a result of trauma or disease.

Body ideal is part of an individual's sense of ideal self. This is likely to be gender- and age-specific and is also influenced by social norms that define appropriate size, shape and contours. In Britain, women's magazines provide a lot of information about appropriate body shape, size and colour, for example urging women to be slim, sun-tanned or have large breasts. A brief look at a history of fashion book will show how women's, and to a lesser extent men's, ideal body shapes have varied over time. There are also cultural variations in what is considered desirable.

Formation of a personal body ideal involves a process of comparison between perceptions of one's real body, cultural norms, and perceptions of one's reference group (see above). If the ideal body image is very different from the perceived reality of the body, the person may feel very dissatisfied.

Janice is approaching the menopause. At one time, a woman aged 50 was considered old, and dressed and acted accordingly. Nowadays, cultural norms for the ideal body have changed. Janice has a friend in her late 50s who wears tight trousers with long boots and is seeking cosmetic surgery to make her look younger. Janice has already started dyeing her hair and is determined to look as young as possible.

Body presentation includes the characteristic ways in which the body moves or functions in social situations. This includes gestures and physical actions; even very subtle facial movements or hand gestures convey information to people. This is called **non-verbal communication**. Some 'innate' responses, such as smiling or laughing when we are happy, are shared by all people. Other 'acquired' responses, such as hand waving, nodding or winking, mean different things to different cultural groups. We acquire these behaviours through a process of socialization and use them in a largely unconscious way. In fact, we may feel very awkward if we try to suppress innate or acquired behaviours. When these responses are changed by a disease process it can make interactions appear very difficult and uncomfortable. For example, someone who has Parkinson's disease may show very little facial movement and, to others, this can make them seem quite disinterested in what is going on around them.

Having a body that does not conform to the norms of a society or reference group can cause psychological harm. Children appear particularly quick to detect differences, even in such minor deviations as being short or having red hair. Those with disabilities or disfigurements are often subject to taunts, stares or discrimination. Changes in body image can also have a distressing effect on relatives or carers. For example, one of the worst aspects of caring for someone with advanced cancer is the change brought about by cachexia (wasting). Sometimes the body changes that result from disease are so severe that relatives may fail to recognize them as the person they love. Mental changes can be equally distressing.

Ted's friend, Dick, has a wife with Alzheimer's disease. It has got so bad that she no longer remembers her own son or daughter. Dick is very upset that the women he once loved has changed so much. It often feels like he is living with a stranger.

Social roles

According to Goffman (1959), an important part of the self concept is determined by the social roles people play. Everyone plays a large number of social roles, at the same as well as different points in their lives.

Anna has various roles as friend, daughter, aunt, nurse, part-time barmaid, and girlfriend. Some of these are a familiar, taken-for-granted part of her life, though recently she returned home and found that her role as daughter had changed because of her increased independence and confidence. However, she is still learning her role as nurse and frequently faces feelings of uncertainty and self-consciousness.

A period of 'socialization' is required before roles become internalized and taken for granted.

Goffman's dramaturgical model

Like Shakespeare, Goffman likened the experience of living to a drama that takes place in the theatre of everyday life. Thus our social roles may be seen as the roles in a play and the social environment the stage set. He suggested that any one person will have available to them a number of different social roles according to the setting they are in at the time. He noted that we all use 'props' to support our various roles. You will observe how doctors use a stethoscope not just as a clinical tool but to define their medical role. As nurses extend their role, you may observe them using the stethoscope or other pieces of equipment in the same way. The way we play our roles depends to a great extent on social expectations. Each member of the health and social care profession has a role that is defined largely by public expectation, often informed by films or soap operas rather than real life.

Goffman proposed that the performance of a particular role is appropriate only in certain social situations. For example, we may be kind and gentle with patients, but noisy or comical with friends. Thus our identity is largely determined by the social situation we are in at the time. People can cause offence if they misjudge social roles. For example, care staff risk offending an older gentleman if they refer to him as 'grandpa' when he feels that is an inappropriate role for him in the context of his illness.

> When Jo was young, he knew a boy called Matt who was eventually diagnosed as having Asperger's syndrome (American Psychiatric Association, 2000). Matt was unable to read social cues or understand accepted rules of social interaction (see Chapter 6). He had difficulty making appropriate eye contact and failed to 'read' social signals. He would interrupt other children's conversations and games and fail to recognize why they got annoyed with him. This meant that most other children did not want him for a friend and he became socially excluded.

Most people learn the rules of social engagement automatically as part of normal development. Where this fails, it is important to teach these skills from an early age in much the same way that a child can learn to play the piano (Stewart, 2002). Failure to do so can lead to social isolation.

Impression management

Goffman outlined how we use various props to help sustain our roles and present the image we wish to portray. He termed this 'impression management'. Clothes, hairstyle, make-up, perfume and mobile phone are all examples of the props we use to portray the public image we wish to present. The doctor's stethoscope and white coat are part of the props used to create the image of the doctor. In fact, the performance of some 'bogus' doctors has been so convincing that it has taken a long time before their lack of medical knowledge or expertise has exposed them.

Each profession has its own set of props and behaviour into which newcomers are initiated and socialized. These are often learned by modelling (copying) rather than formal instruction. However, we eventually learn to regulate and modify our own behaviour as necessary (Chapter 4). Role development is a process of learning how to look and how to behave, testing and readjusting the role. For example, each health professional develops a distinctive role that involves certain norms and expectations of social behaviour.

Changing roles

It can be quite difficult to make the transition between roles we are expected to play at different points in the lifespan.

During Janice's lifetime, she has had to adjust from being single to being married and becoming a parent. She adapted from being the mother of young children to having adolescent offspring to being alone with her husband again. She was a carer to her mother-in-law, Laura, and now has to care for Ted. Her role has changed to chief wage-earner since Mark retired. Her role as wife and lover has changed over the years, particularly since Mark's health has deteriorated.

Illness and disability interfere expectedly with the ability of the individual to engage in pleasurable activities or continue in previous social roles. People who have lived independent lives or cared for others suddenly become dependent. Social roles are an integral part of our sense of self and enforced restrictions are an important source of loss of identity, resulting in psychological harm.

Everyone holds some kind of mental representation of themselves. This is referred to as the self concept or self schema. A schema refers to the integration of complex information to form a coherent and relatively stable internal image or mental representation (Chapters 3 and 5). Some people have a unified self schema and think of themselves as having the same attributes in every situation and in every role. Others have several clearly differentiated self schemas and think of themselves as having quite different attributes in different roles and situations. In an early study, Linville (1987) found that people vary in their ability to perceive themselves differently in different situations. Linville showed that having a complex self schema that varies in different situations appears to make people more adaptive and resilient to stress-related illness and depression. However, many of the difficulties people have in adjusting their roles following illness are caused not by personal strengths or weaknesses, but by the attitudes of others.

Stigma

Goffman (1963) introduced the concept of stigma to refer to a visible sign that distinguishes an individual or group. The concept is important in psychology because stigmas lead to negative perceptions and behaviours by others. Goffman described three types of stigma:

- Moral behaviour or attributes that violate cultural or social values.
- Tribal features or adornments which signal group membership.
- Physical deviations from normal appearance which may be interpreted as deformity or disfigurement.

'Moral stigma' refers to attributes of the individual that are regarded as morally reprehensible in a particular culture at a particular time. Certain body characteristics may be stigmatized. For example, children who are obese are often taunted as lazy or clumsy by their classmates. Behaviours may be stigmatized. For example, smoking has come to be regarded by many as unacceptable in public places. The debate about whether smokers should be offered heart surgery could be said to illustrate stigmatizing attitudes on the part of health professionals.

'Tribal stigma' refers to marks or adornments that signal group membership and status. The wearing of head coverings by Muslim or Orthodox Jewish women is an example of this. In health care we need to respect the wish to continue wearing these adornments in hospital. For example, we do not normally expect married women to remove their wedding rings before surgery.

'Physical stigma' refers to alterations in the body or in bodily functions that mark people out from the rest. These may be immediately identifiable things such as an amputated leg or scarred face. Some changes in function are not readily identifiable but can have an incapacitating effect. For example, incontinence is an important reason why some older people refuse to leave their homes. Changes in body odour, such as the smell of a leg ulcer, can also serve to make people feel stigmatized. Some conditions like epilepsy or HIV are not readily apparent to an outside observer. But people with these conditions have to make difficult choices about disclosure. If they tell other people, they risk stigmatization. If they do not, they have to live with the fear of being found out.

A stigma is essentially an identity acquired from the reactions of other people. Once a stigmatizing label has been attached to an individual, it is difficult to remove.

A classic study by Rosenhan (1973), 'On being sane in insane places', illustrated how a diagnosis of mental illness, once established, can be difficult to shake off. In Rosenhan's study, several 'normal' people, including a psychologist, paediatrician and psychiatrist, worker and housewife presented themselves at a psychiatric clinic complaining of hearing voices. During their assessment, all details of their stories were correct apart from their claims to hear voices. All were diagnosed as having major mental illness, in most cases schizophrenia, and were admitted to hospital. Following admission, they stopped complaining about the voices, but in most cases it took several weeks to convince staff that they were in remission and well enough to be discharged. Only fellow inmates were suspicious about their true identities. This study was later the subject of the film *One Flew Over the Cuckoo's Nest*.

Mental health problems have long been stigmatized by the public, with the result that those who have suffered an episode of depression or other serious mental illness may find it difficult to obtain work. Cancer was until recently a stigmatized disease, to be talked about in hushed tones. According to Goffman, stigmatized people have to negotiate a new identity and may use a number of tactics to do this. One is to mix only with other people who share similar attributes. For example, some deaf people who use sign language may feel more comfortable in social situations where signing is the dominant communication system. They do not need to explain to others that they are deaf nor are they stared at and made to feel abnormal when they are signing. It is often difficult for parents of deaf children to know how much to encourage their children to form relationships with other deaf people or how much they should be helped to integrate into the hearing world. Other ways of dealing with an obvious stigma include preparing explanations to share with others; ignoring the disability and hoping that everyone else does as well; and using humour to avoid embarrassment.

The stigma of facial disfigurement

Facial appearance is particularly important to the development of a positive body image. Physical attractiveness is known to be a significant component in social interaction. Parents are often very distressed by the appearance of a baby with a cleft lip and/or palate and may, as a result, find it difficult to form a close attachment to the baby. Seeing another baby who has been successfully treated can be very reassuring to the parents at an early stage. Research suggests that fears about the social consequences of facial disfigurement are well founded.

> Houston and Bull (1994) conducted a series of studies that involved marking the face of a normal individual with a port wine type stain. The 'stigmatized individual' then took up a seat in a railway carriage while an observer recorded the behaviour of the other passengers. They found that when the subject sat with the marked side of the face towards an adjacent empty seat, people tended to avoid sitting there until the other seats were occupied.

More recent work by Coull (2003) highlighted similar and worse personal experiences reported by burns patients. It appears that people with physical differences, whether congenital or acquired, are probably quite right in fearing that other people will react differently and hold negative attitudes towards them. As a result, they need to learn how to deal with being stared at, ignored or avoided and health professionals need to know how best to help them deal with such situations. Failure to do this may result in social withdrawal and have serious adverse effects on their quality of life. A useful review of the issues, together with advice for professionals on how to help people with disfigurement, is provided by Newell (2002a, 2002b).

Attitudes

Attitudes are subjective evaluations that predispose people to behave towards an object or person in a positive or negative way. The object may be a health-related topic (see Chapter 8). But it is commonly another person or group of people. Attitudes are generally conceptualized as consisting of three classes of response:

- Cognitive (beliefs about the object);
- Affective (a positive or negative evaluative feeling towards the object);
- Behavioural (actions directed at the object).

Attitudes are culturally shaped through formal socialization processes, including child-rearing, schooling and professional training. They may also be the product of identification with social groupings such as religious, kinship or friendship groups. These groups exert strong influence or 'peer pressure' on the behaviour of group members. Conformity to 'social norms' laid down by the group is very strong and attitudes towards 'others' may be hostile (Chapter 6). Negative attitudes are an important part of stigmatization, stereotyping and prejudice.

Stereotyping, prejudice and discrimination

Stereotyping is a convenient form of shared schema for describing and categorizing people. It involves attaching attributes to an individual on the basis of their group membership. Sociologists refer to this process as 'labelling'. It draws on certain salient characteristics that usually have some foundation in fact or experience. Some categories, such as personality types or diagnostic categories, are determined by objective assessment using scientifically valid and reliable instruments. They are intended to assist with psychological or medical treatment, but even these can lead to stereotyping if the group label takes precedence over individualized care planning. Most stereotypes, however, are based on folklore, lay assumptions or uninformed biased attitudes. These often involve characteristics that are exaggerated and generalized at the expense of individual attributes. Stereotypes are often based upon features such as age or gender, ethnic, national or regional characteristics, personal appearance or ethnic origin. Some stereotypes are positive, but many are negative. For example, it is often said that people with red hair have fiery tempers, Scottish people are mean, and fat people are lazy. These assumptions are usually untrue when applied to individuals and can be very damaging. Negative stereotypes lead to prejudice and discrimination and may become self-fulfilling prophecies.

The negative effects of stereotyping are to be found in prejudice and discrimination. Prejudice refers to the combination of negative beliefs and attitudes towards an individual or group, and discrimination refers to the negative behaviour associated with prejudice. Many beliefs about others are based on limited knowledge of their social grouping. For example, it is not unusual to see people grouped together on the basis of age, gender, social class or medical condition, and then treated accordingly. These beliefs and expectations can and do change the ways that people behave, and this has important implications for those working in health care settings.

The self-fulfilling prophecy

The effects of expectations were well illustrated in a series of social psychology experiments conducted by Rosenthal and colleagues in the 1960s.

Rosenthal and Jacobson (1968) examined the effect of expectation on children in a classic experiment on teacher expectations in the classroom. The result became known as the 'Pygmalion effect'. At the beginning of the school year, students took an IQ test and were then randomly labelled as either clever or ordinary. The teacher was told to expect that the clever ones would make rapid progress. Students took a further IQ test at the end of the year and the 'clever' students were found to have made greater gains in IQ than the ordinary students. This demonstrated clearly that students who are expected to do well, do better, but why? Observations suggested that students labelled as clever received more attention, more encouragement and more positive feedback from the teacher than the other pupils.

In the field of health care, the self-fulfilling prophecy may be an important predictor of patients' behaviour. The expectations of health professionals are often influenced by personal observations or value judgements recorded in, or implicit from, patients' records.

Lillian had previously had little contact with doctors when she was referred to the hospital for investigation. Her general practitioner was sympathetic and wrote in the referral letter 'This pleasant lady . . .'. She found the staff very sympathetic and helpful. But the lady she sat next to in the waiting room had quite a different experience. She had a thick set of notes that catalogued a series of health problems that had not responded to treatment. She felt that none of the staff seemed interested in her any more.

Factors that influence our expectations include 'stigma' such as age or gender, appearance, the way in which an individual dresses, their accent, the questions they ask, and their illness behaviours (Chapter 4).

In the early 1970s, Stockwell (1984) first reported the findings of a classic nursing study which sought to identify the characteristics of 'unpopular' patients. She found factors that accounted for lack of popularity with nursing staff included physical features, physical defects, nationality, length of stay and the need for time-consuming care. Other factors have been identified as complaining (Walker *et al.* 1990) and social worth or value (Johnson and Webb 1995). Taylor (1979) observed that 'good patient' behaviour involves being quiet, passive and undemanding. But these characteristics may also be indicative of dependence and depression, rather than confidence and self-management. Being passive is not conducive to the achievement of a 'patient–professional partnership' or to becoming an 'expert patient'. Yet those who are vocal about expressing their needs may become unpopular with care staff.

It is not just patients who are expected to conform to certain stereotypes. Each profession appears to hold a stereotypical set of expectations about members of other professions (Chapter 6). This can interfere with interprofessional working, to the detriment of patient care.

Attribution theory

Attribution theory is a dominant theory in social psychology. It refers to processes by which people understand relationships between cause and effect, and how they make judgements about responsibility and blame. Based on the work of Kurt Lewin in the 1930s, attribution theory was proposed by Fritz Heider in the 1940s and developed further by Harold Kelley in the 1970s (Hewstone 1989). It is based on the premise that people have an intrinsic need to understand cause–effect relationships.

Unlike other theories of decision-making, attribution theory recognizes that most events take place in a social setting where there needs to be some way of deciding who or what was responsible for what occurred. Attribution theory, as applied in health care, proposes that decisions about causality take place on three separate dimensions:

- locus   internal – external (self or other);
- stability   stable – unstable (always or just on this occasion);
- globality   global – specific (in all situations, or just in this situation).

The internal–external dimension is usually referred to as **locus of control** (Chapter 4). The theory is illustrated in the following example:

Anna failed her first examination. As a result, she may decide that she is just no good at examinations. This involves an internal, stable and global attribution for failure. On the other hand, she may decide that on this occasion the paper was an unfair test of her knowledge (external, unstable, specific attributions). Or she may decide that on this occasion, she did not work hard enough (internal, unstable, specific attributions).

Different sets of attributions can have important implications for future actions. If Anna makes internal, stable and global attributions for failure (I am always a stupid person), she will feel that she is a failure and may become depressed. If she makes external, unstable and specific attributions (it is their fault for setting such a silly test on this occasion), she may blame the module leader. This will help her to feel better about her failure, but will not encourage her to work harder for her resit paper. On the other hand, if she makes internal, unstable and specific attributions (it was my own fault on this occasion), she is well placed to address her failure and make sure that she passes next time.

There is good evidence in health care that internal locus of control is associated with better health outcomes in a variety of situations (Chapters 7 and 8).

The fundamental attribution error

Attribution theory helps us understand how we make judgements about the actions of others. If someone is anxious, we may attribute their anxiety to their personality (internal, stable and global attributions). Or we may, if we have taken a little time to find out the reasons for their anxiety, attribute this to specific worries or concerns about their illness or what is happening at home (external, unstable, specific attributions). The attributions we make about responses such as anxiety will have important implications for the way we respond to others. Quite often, we draw on stereotypes (negative, stable and global attributions) when making these judgements.

It appears that the attributions we make about our own successes or failures are often quite different from those we make about others. For example:

- If I make a mistake, I am most likely to believe it is because I was given the wrong information.
- If somebody else makes a similar mistake, I am more likely to believe it is because they are stupid.
- If I am anxious about an illness symptom, I am likely to believe there must be a physical cause, even if the doctor cannot find one.
- If a patient is worried about an illness symptom for which there is no apparent cause, health professionals may believe that he or she is a hypochondriac.

The pervasive tendency to make external, unstable and specific attributions about our own actions, but internal, stable and global attributions about the actions of others is termed the **fundamental attribution error** (Ross 1977, cited in Brehm *et al.* 2002). The fundamental attribution error has been defined as one of the most potent sources of human error and is an important reason for victim-blaming.

> Anna was working alongside a junior doctor who wrote up the wrong dose of drug for a patient. The staff nurse gave the drug before noticing the error. Luckily the patient was unharmed. The junior doctor was disciplined for his mistake, but it probably happened because he was tired and distracted by too many other demands.

In the case of mistakes, it is common for organizations to seek someone to blame, so that they can be disciplined. In reality, it is often a system failure, such as inadequate information or resources, that causes the error. The Department of Health has recognized this as an important cause of persistent medical error and has attempted to introduce a 'no blame' culture into the National Health Service. But the fundamental attribution error is difficult to change.

Trait theory

One of the reasons why we have given little space in this book to the topic of personality is that the inappropriate use of personality labels in health care is an important source of the fundamental attribution error. The identification and use of personality typologies in the absence of a formal training and adequate patient assessment can be dangerous. In the field of mental health, personality traits are often measured as part of a detailed assessment. But in general health care, personality traits are often assigned in the absence of proper assessment.

A trait is a relatively stable set of individual characteristics that include patterns of thought, adjustment and behaviour that are partly inherited, strongly influenced by experiences during childhood, and to some extent modified through adult experiences. Personality and intelligence are examples of such traits. The extent to which inheritance (nature) and child-rearing practices (nurture) influence intelligence and personality traits remains a matter of considerable debate within the scientific community, where it is commonly referred to as the nature–nurture debate.

> The relative contribution of nature versus nurture has been examined through the comparative study of monozygotic (identical) and dizygotic (non-identical) twins. Monozytogic (MZ) twins share identical genetic material, whereas dizygotic (DZ) twins do not. Twin studies normally

compared MZ and DZ twins brought up together with those adopted separately. Borkenau *et al.* (2001) confirmed findings of previous studies that about 40% of personality is genetically determined, and the remaining 60% environmentally determined. Of this 60%, he estimated that 25% was due to shared environment (most of which is likely to be in the parental home), and 35% to non-shared environmental influences.

The names most commonly associated with the measurement of personality are Raymond Cattell and Hans Eysenck. Cattell produced a multi-dimensional measure of personality consisting of 16 traits or personality factors, called the 16 PF. Eysenck, who worked at the Maudsley Hospital in the UK, is particularly well known for his work on the dimensions of extroversion, neuroticism and psychoticism, which are measured using the Eysenck Personality Inventory (EPI). Perhaps the most important of Eysenck's propositions was that extroversion and neuroticism are biologically determined.

The personality measure now in most common use in health psychology is the 'Big Five', which measures the following five traits (Costa and McCrae 1992):

- neuroticism   anxious, tense, worrying, unstable
- extroversion   active, assertive, enthusiastic, outgoing, talkative
- agreeableness   appreciative, forgiving, generous, kind, trusting
- conscientiousness   efficient, organized, reliable, responsible, thorough
- openness   artistic, curious, imaginative, insightful
  (or creativity)

Each of these traits lies at one end of a **bipolar** dimension, and an individual may score anywhere on each of the following dimensions:

- neurotic   versus   emotionally stable;
- extrovert   versus   introvert (reserved);
- agreeable   versus   antagonistic;
- conscientious   versus   disorganized;
- open   versus   closed.

Stability and change in personality

Debate about the stability and change of personality beyond childhood has been vigorous. Early researchers claimed that personality does not change, while subsequent researchers claimed that there were changes in personality over time, but that this was a function of maturation. For example, Costa and McCrae (1992) found that extroversion, openness, and neuroticism declined with age, while conscientiousness and agreeableness increased. Longitudinal studies suggest a level of consistency in personality throughout life, due mainly to genetic factors and parental influence.

But there are also maturational changes resulting from life experiences such as mothering, middle age and getting older. For example, Srivastava *et al.* (2003) conducted a cross-sectional internet survey of adults aged 21–60, using the Big Five personality measure. Conscientiousness and agreeableness increased throughout early and middle adulthood at varying rates, while neuroticism declined among women but did not change among men. Helson *et al.* (2002) found considerable individual variability in personality change over time and confirmed personality changes in response to time of life and cultural climate.

Evidence from a wide range of studies appears to indicate that we are born with distinctive personalities, but there is still a lot of room for change. Our personalities develop during our formative years and continue to change in adulthood in response to age-related and culturally determined demands. But there are also considerable individual differences in the ways that our personalities change in response to life experiences. This suggests that it can be dangerous for health care professionals to believe that an individual's personality tells them anything meaningful about the way they are likely to respond to a particular illness or event.

Personality and physical health

An important reason for measuring personality traits is that it is believed they predict adjustment to different aspects of life.

Friedman (2000) reviewed links between personality and physical health, based on a seven-decade longitudinal study. He offered three possible theoretical explanations for links between personality and health:

1. Certain personality types may be associated with physiological mechanisms that lead to certain diseases, for example coronary heart disease and cancer.
2. Personality traits may set a trajectory towards health or disease. For example, those who are more sociable may develop better support networks than others.
3. Personality may be associated with certain motivational forces that draw people towards rebellion or risk, including substance use.

Friedman examined these explanations in relation to three of the Big Five personality types: sociability (extroversion), conscientiousness and neuroticism. Conscientiousness was found to be a predictor of good health, possibly because conscientious people are likely to smoke less, moderate their alcohol consumption, have greater work and social stability, and adhere to medical treatments where necessary.

Vollrath and Torgersen (2000) confirmed that a combination of low neuroticism and high conscientiousness is associated with favourable health. This means that those who are emotionally unstable and use passive strategies are more susceptible to stress and stress-related illness. These researchers described the effects of extroversion on health as ambiguous. Extroverts are often optimistic and have good support networks, but are also high risk-takers and more likely to engage in unhealthy behaviours such as drinking and smoking. Therefore the negative effects tend to cancel out the positive effects.

Friedman (2000) concluded that there is little evidence to support the notion of a disease-prone personality. Certain people are more likely to take up unhealthy habits, exhibit unbalanced emotional and physiological responses, and experience unsupportive social environments that overall are conducive to poor health. He argued that these causal processes, rather than personality *per se*, need to be taken into account when offering health advice.

Certain patterns of thought and behaviour, such as self-efficacy and locus of control (Chapter 4), have been shown to influence health-related ways of coping with difficult life changes or events. But these have been shown to be amenable to change and are not considered to be personality traits.

Personality and mental health

The relationship between neuroticism and anxiety-related disorders is self-evident. Neuroticism refers to emotional instability and it is no surprise that mental health problems are commonly associated with having a neurotic personality.

Goodwin *et al.* (2002) set out to determine the relationship between personality factors and the use of mental health services among adults living in New York. They found that neuroticism was associated with an increased likelihood of service utilization. Conscientiousness and extroversion were associated with decreased likelihood of utilization. This appears to suggest, perhaps not surprisingly, that reserved, passive people who are emotionally unstable and lack a sense of commitment are more likely to require treatment for mental health problems.

Problems with personality theory

There is little doubt that all people have certain characteristics that tend to endure during the course of their lives. Patterns of neural response and behaviour, present from birth, undoubtedly influence the different ways in which parents and others respond to the growing child. This explains why two children reared in similar ways by the same parents can turn out to be very different adults. There is no doubt that commonalities in the ageing process and cultural demands and expectations at different points in the lifespan influence common patterns of change over time. But the evidence, such as it is, indicates that there is a large amount of individual variation.

This suggests that health care professionals must be very careful not to use stereotypical explanations when working with individuals who experience mental or physical illness or other life-changing experiences. If we believe that the way an individual behaves is a consequence of their personality, we may accept that they are unlikely to change. This can lead us to do nothing and our negative expectations may become to be a self-fulfilling prophecy. However, if we believe, as do humanist psychologists (Chapter 1), in the potential for human growth, we will endeavour to find ways to encourage and facilitate positive change and adaptation.

Summary of key points

- Much of what we think of as our 'self' is defined by the ways that other people respond to us.
- Looks are important. Looking or behaving differently, whether through disability or choice, can lead to avoidance or labelling as 'different' or deviant.
- The labels we attach to ourselves and others can become self-fulfilling prophecies.
- If we treat people positively, they are more likely to respond in a positive way. It is never too late to change.
- Listening to people's stories is informative and can have therapeutic value.
- The labelling of people according to personality traits or types may lead to the fundamental attribution error, in which their behaviour is attributed to personal characteristics rather than to situational factors.

Further reading

Brewer, M.B. and Hewstone, M. (2004) *Self and Social Identity*. Oxford: Blackwell.

Goffman, E. (1959) *The Presentation of Self in Everyday Life*. London: Penguin.

Goffman, E. (1963) *Stigma: Notes on the Management of Spoiled Identity*. Harmondsworth: Penguin.

Johnson, M. and Webb, C. (1995) Rediscovering the unpopular patients: the concept of social judgement. *Journal of Advanced Nursing* 21(3), 466–74.

Stockwell, F. (1984) *The Unpopular Patient*. London: Croom Helm.

CHAPTER THREE

MEMORY, UNDERSTANDING AND INFORMATION-GIVING

- What influences *what* we remember?
- What influences *how* much we remember?
- Why do we forget?
- How is our understanding influenced by our existing knowledge?
- What are the main causes of memory loss and confusion in older people?
- How can we give information in a way that improves memory and understanding?
- What are the best ways of breaking bad news?

Memory

Memory involves receiving, processing, encoding, storing and retrieving information. Memory loss or forgetting may occur at any stage, although most information appears to be lost at the receiving, processing and retrieval stages. In this section, these issues are explored and the implications for patient care examined.

To illustrate some of these points, we have linked them to a situation in which Lillian is being given the results of a biopsy she recently had taken from a lump in her neck.

Doctor: Well, Lillian, the tests show that you have a type of cancerous growth called a lymphoma. This type of tumour normally responds well to treatment. We will get you into hospital next week to remove the lump and then organize some follow-up treatment in the form of chemotherapy.

Arousal and attention

In order to receive any type of information, we must pay attention to it. In other words, the information must stimulate our interest and arrest our attention. This implies a state of arousal, which refers to the arousal of the autonomic nervous system and release of adrenalin that prepares the body for action. Based on research over many years, it is well established that cognitive performance, including memory, is related to our level of arousal. But this relationship is not linear. There appears to be an inverse U relationship between arousal and cognitive performance which is termed the Yerkes–Dodson law (see Figure 3.1.) Since arousal is frequently associated with feelings of anxiety, the Yerkes–Dodson law applies equally to levels of anxiety. This is explained below.

A low level of arousal reflects a state of apathy or disinterest. If Lillian is in this state, she may not be taking the situation seriously and is unlikely to be attending to the information being presented. Therefore her memory encoding is likely to be minimal and she will be unable to recall what she was told.

An extremely high level of arousal is associated with a high level of anxiety or panic. If this were the case, Lillian would probably be unable to attend properly to any type of cognitive task and her memory encoding is likely to be poor. Her attention may focus solely on the most salient aspect of the information received, and this is not necessarily the main point the doctor wished to convey.

The best cognitive performance is obtained if Lillian is aroused, slightly anxious, alert and her attention clearly focused upon the task in hand. This would enable her to concentrate on and encode what was being said and to recall more accurately the information she was given. This highlights the importance of noting the patient's emotional state when trying to give important information. Time needs to be taken to listen to and calm someone who is highly anxious, or alert someone of the importance of an issue, if they are totally unconcerned.

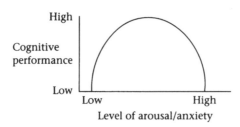

Figure 3.1   The Yerkes–Dodson law of the relationship between arousal and cognitive performance.

Short-term memory

It is generally accepted that there are two types of memory storage: short-term and long-term memory. Short-term memory is also referred to as working memory since remembering at this level is an active and conscious process. Research by Ebbinghaus and Wundt in the nineteenth century, using nonsense syllables, showed that the capacity of short-term memory was in the region of seven digits. Miller (1956) confirmed that short-term memory has a processing capacity that is limited to 7±2 bits of information. The combination of seven letters and numbers in the British car number plate was determined by this psychological research. But a 'bit' is not the same thing as a letter or number. You will note that it is much easier to remember a number plate such as LIM1T, which effectively reduces five digits to one meaningful chunk or 'bit' of information. In contrast, in the number plate that reads NMG3P, each of the five digits is a separate, unrelated bit of information.

How many separate bits or chunks of information are commonly given to patients during a single consultation? In the short extract from Lillian's consultation, it is possible to identify at least nine separate bits of information that make it unlikely that Lillian will remember all of it:

Doctor: Well, Lillian, the tests show that you have

1. a type of cancerous growth
2. called a lymphoma.
3. This type of tumour
4. normally responds well to treatment.
5. We will get you into hospital
6. next week
7. to remove the lump
8. and then organize some follow-up treatment
9. in the form of chemotherapy.

The holding of information in short-term memory, and its transfer to long-term memory, are facilitated by repetition and association. If we wish to remember a telephone number, we keep repeating it until it has 'sunk in'. If we are distracted during this process, we often have to start all over again. When we are given a series of important items of information in a short space of time, there is no opportunity to repeat all of it. This helps to explain why much of it is promptly lost. Lillian's consultation is time-limited and is likely to cover a lot of information, most of which will never reach her long- term memory.

It is possible to improve memory by using memory-enhancing devices such as mnemonics. Mnemonic techniques are useful ways of organizing discrete bits of information into a meaningful chunk. For example, if I wish to remember the number plate NMG3P, I might make up a little saying, such as 'No Man Goes (for) 3p'. This would be even more memorable if it was accompanied by a visual image of a car at a tollgate. Mnemonics are commonly used to assist remembering medical information. For example, a common mnemonic for remembering the first letters of the names of the 12 cranial nerves was: 'On Old Olympic's Towering Tops, A Fin And German Viewed Some Hops'.

In the case of treatment regimes, patients could be encouraged to repeat their instructions several times and relate them to daily events, such as meals, in order to retain the information. When trying to remember which tablet is for what, 'white for water, blue for blood, yellow for yawning (sleep)' might prove memorable if the colours of the tablets were obliging enough to conform to this mnemonic. It is probably best if patients invent their own, but they may need some encouragement to do so. Some people prefer verbal mnemonics while others prefer visual ones. Of course, the best way of ensuring that something is not forgotten is to write it down. It would be helpful if Lillian was given written information about her condition and treatment so that she could take away and read it at her leisure.

Familiarity, salience and selective attention

Even when people are attending to what is being said, their attention will tend to focus upon things that are familiar or important to them. In other words, people tend to pay attention to what they know about or expect to hear and not necessarily to the things that health professionals feel are important. In Lillian's case, the salient aspects of information are highlighted in italic below:

> Doctor: Well, Lillian, the tests show that you have a type of *cancer* called a lymphoma. This type of tumour normally responds well to treatment. We will get you into *hospital* next week for an *operation* to remove the lump and then organize some follow-up treatment in the form of *chemotherapy*.

Lillian is likely to hear certain key words during her consultation, of which 'cancer' is probably the most important. This may interfere with her ability to hear other important details, such as 'the tumour normally responds well to treatment'. Furthermore, you may have noticed that Lillian's problem is referred to in four different ways: cancer, lymphoma, tumour, lump. Lillian may or may not realize that these terms refer to the same thing.

Selective attention is an important problem in relation to health promotion. Eiser and Gentle (1989) noted that there is good evidence that the people most likely to attend to health messages are those who are already following the health advice being given. This is because the information reinforces their existing attitudes and behaviour. Those whose behaviour is contrary to the advice being given tend to disregard it as irrelevant.

Primacy and recency effects

When people are given several pieces of information in sequence, they are most likely to remember the thing they were told first (the primacy effect) and the thing they were told last (the recency effect), and to forget most of the rest. One of the reasons for this is that they have more opportunity to mentally rehearse these items. In the case of Lillian's information, this means that she is most likely to remember the fact that she has cancer and will have to have chemotherapy.

Doctor: Well, Lillian, the tests show that you have

1. a type of *cancer*ous growth
2. called a lymphoma.
3. This type of tumour
4. normally responds well to treatment.
5. We will get you into hospital
6. next week
7. to remove the lump
8. and then organize some follow-up treatment
9. in the form of *chemotherapy*.

Conveying useful information

Health professionals can use memory research to try to ensure that they give the most important information first and repeat it last. Thus if the doctor really wishes to convey to Lillian the good news that her lump is likely to respond to treatment, it would be better to approach this by reordering the sequence of the information given to Lillian:

Doctor: Well, Lillian,

1. *I am pleased to tell you that your tests indicate that you have something that is likely to respond well to treatment.*
   [Pause]
2. The lump is a form of cancer
3. called a lymphoma.
4. We will need to bring you into hospital
5. next week
6. to remove the lump
7. and then give you some further treatment
8. in the form of chemotherapy.
9. *Fortunately, the outcomes of this treatment are good.*
   [Pause]

Presenting positive information first and repeating it last emphasizes the likelihood of a positive outcome. The pauses also allow time for important information to be attended to and facilitate its transfer from short-term into long-term memory. In this case, Lillian is much more likely to go away feeling positive about her results. Even where an outcome is not so positive, this approach can be used to highlight the fact that everything possible will be done to ensure the well-being of the individual.

Long-term memory

Long-term memory has been the subject of much research and theory development in psychology, assisted more recently by the introduction of brain scanning and imaging techniques. Once transferred from short-term to long-term memory, memories are stored in the brain according to series of complex linkages between language, meanings, emotions, images, sounds and responses that are still not fully understood. Long-term memory is normally divided into three distinct types:

- Procedural memory is concerned with motor skills, rules, habits or sequences, as in riding a bike.
- Semantic memory is concerned with general knowledge, or knowledge of facts, and is heavily dependent on language.
- Episodic or autobiographical memory is concerned with memory of events from the past and is strongly associated with sensory images.

Procedural memory is related to habit formation (see conditioning, Chapter 4), and is extremely enduring. Semantic memory may be subject to interference and is commonly affected during dementia. Autobiographical memory tends also to be very enduring and it is common to find that even older people with severe Alzheimer's disease are able to retain vivid memories of certain salient or transformatory events from their past. This may be because emotionally arousing events are more easily or strongly embedded within our long-term memories and become more memorable. McGaugh (2003) reminds us that autobiographical memories connect our past to our present and help us to predict the future. This aspect of memory is fundamental to our sense of self (Chapter 2) and to the way we cope with loss and other stressful events (Chapters 5 and 7).

Understanding

Remembering is not the same as understanding. For example, Anna was able to recall the list of cranial nerves for her examination, but found it difficult to organize and present them in a coherent way because she had not fully understood their functions. Lay people are often disadvantaged in health care settings by their limited knowledge and understanding of their bodies (see also Chapter 5 on children's understandings). It is only fairly recently in evolutionary history that adult humans have had much idea about the nature and function of internal organs, and many adults today have little idea about how their bodies actually work. As health professionals, we should not take for granted that patients understand the names, functions and locations of essential organs, or that they necessarily wish to know.

Adults may sometimes suffer unnecessary illness or disability as a result of erroneous beliefs about their bodies and body functions. For example, people with back pain frequently avoid activity or exercise in the mistaken belief that hurt equals harm. The emphasis during the latter part of the twentieth century on 'slipped disc' as a cause of back pain has led many people to believe that further movement could lead to permanent damage. Doctors reinforced this belief by wrongly recommending bed rest for back pain. In fact, most back pain is caused by damage to the muscles or ligaments that support the spine. There is actually little correlation between the changes to the spine seen on X-rays or magnetic resonance imaging (MRI) scans and the amount of pain experienced. Most of these changes are a normal result of the ageing process and were present before the injury took place. Therefore, in the vast majority of cases of back pain, it is the fear that pain signals harm, and not the injury itself, that causes disability (Vlaeyen and Linton 2000).

Mental schemas and scripts

Recent memory research has focused upon the fact that individuals tend to encode information in relation to their own framework of understanding, which is referred to as a mental schema (schemas were also mentioned in Chapter 2 in relation to the self concept). This explains why familiarity and salience are so important and why attention and memory tend to be selective. Schemas enable us to organize and process large amounts of information, but their existence implies that memory encoding and recall involve a certain amount of selectivity and reconstruction.

A famous experiment by George Bartlett, reported in the 1930s, studied what happens when a complex and mysterious legend or story is passed from one person to another, in the same way as 'Chinese whispers'. He selected a North American folk tale, 'The War of the Ghosts', that contained a number of features that were strange and difficult to make sense of for those in twentieth-century western cultures. He found that the story changed in certain predictable ways as it was passed on. The story became shorter, more coherent and more conventional, to fit in with common cultural ways of understanding. The study is easy to replicate and demonstrates that while distinctive and familiar events are retained, recall changes to fit in with the framework of understanding of the individual.

Bartlett's work highlighted that memory schemas are strongly influenced by shared social and cultural understandings. When a patient is given medical information by word of mouth, they tell their friends and relatives, who tell other friends and relatives. The story is simplified in the telling. If this information contains complex terms or relates to unfamiliar procedures, it is perhaps not surprising that important details are changed to fit in with the frame of reference of those giving and receiving the information. It is not unusual for doctors and other health care professionals to note that a patient reports a completely different version of events from the recorded account. This may be because the patient's framework of understanding is different from that of the health professional. It is therefore important to establish the patient's understanding of the situation before and after a consultation. The use of technical or medical jargon, whether spoken or written, compounds this problem since patients will tend to reinterpret something they have fully understood into their own schema (see also Vygotsky's theory of development in Chapter 5).

Mental schemas and autobiographical memories are gaining increasing attention within narrative psychology. Receiving medical information is not just a matter of remembering a list of facts. Finding out that one has a disease may confront the individual with a major sense of biographical disruption (Chapter 2). Therefore, as patients are receiving news about their disease and treatment, they may be trying to make sense of this in the context of their life story.

> When Lillian heard the doctor tell her she had cancer, she started thinking about the much longed-for holiday she was due to go on with a friend in two months' time. It was her first long-distance holiday and she had spent so much time planning and looking forward to it. Logically, her health was far more important, but why this and why now? All she could think about was that it could not possibly be happening to her. Perhaps she would wake up in the morning and find that it was all a bad dream. As she considered this, she realized that she had missed most of what the doctor was saying. She did not like to ask the doctor to repeat it, even when asked if she had understood everything, because the doctor was obviously very busy.

Recognition, false memories and context-specific memories

Recognition is easier than recall because recognition involves a prompt. Recall is a reconstructive process that is subject to a number of external influences. People asked to describe an event often come up with quite different accounts or details. It is relatively easy to 'plant' memories by the use of prompts or probes. This is why interviewing witnesses, especially child witnesses, requires special skills. If you wish to find out what a patient has remembered it is better to ask an open question like 'can you tell me what the doctor said to you last time?' than a closed question like 'do you remember that last time you were told . . .?'.

There have been accusations in the media that psychotherapy may lead to the recovery of false memories about such events as childhood sexual abuse. Memories associated with events that cause emotional arousal are usually better embedded in memory. But, bearing in mind the Yerkes–Dodson law, intense physiological arousal during trauma may eliminate memory processing. Alternatively, clinical psychologists sometimes refer to 'dissociation', which implies that traumatic memories have become cut off from conscious thought as a form of self-protection. Given these different explanations, it is very hard to know if someone has 'recovered' a memory for a real event or one that never actually occurred. In either case, it is important that practitioners do not provide prompts or leading information that can lead to false reconstructions.

Certain memories are context-specific and are aided by a return to the environment or emotional state in which information was originally received. You have probably had an experience where a certain piece of music or smell triggers a forgotten event. Similarly, patients may have entirely forgotten an instruction or piece of advice until returning to the sight and smell of the hospital. Only then do they remember what they should have done, but may be too embarrassed to admit that they did not do it.

Forgetting

Memory loss is rarely due to the decay or loss of memories, but is more often caused by problems in transferring information from short-term memory into long-term memory, or in retrieving information from long-term memory. Recent research by Anderson (2003) suggests that it may be difficult to encode new information that threatens to disrupt existing patterns of belief or ways of behaving. This lends support to Festinger's theory of cognitive dissonance (Chapter 6), but there may also be a structural explanation. De Beni and Palladino (2004) studied short-term memory between the ages of 55 and 75 and found that older people had greater difficulty accommodating new information into their existing memory schemas. This means that when giving patients information it is necessary first to check out their understanding.

> Doctor: Lillian, perhaps you would like to tell me what you understand about what is wrong and what the plan is for your treatment.

It may be that a patient's apparent failure to grasp what they were told is caused by their inability to update existing schemas, or by the threat to their existing belief systems. In such cases, it is best to start with what they already know or believe and build gradually on this, taking account of the coping strategies available to the individual (Chapter 7). This can be demanding in terms of time and patience, but it is pointless for the health professional to try in vain to bombard the patient with advice and instructions that cannot be assimilated.

It is often assumed that older people are less likely to adhere to medication use than younger people because of poorer memory. But this appears to be a stereotypical belief for which there is little evidence:

> Park *et al.* (1999) created an age-stratified profile of individuals with rheumatoid arthritis and studied factors that influenced adherence to medications. They assessed cognitive function, disability, emotional state, lifestyle, and beliefs about the illness. They found that older adults made the fewest adherence errors, and middle-aged adults made the most. Despite strong evidence for normal, age-related, cognitive decline, most older adults had sufficient cognitive function to manage medications. A busy lifestyle was the strongest predictor of non-adherence, and this was more likely to occur in middle life.

Health care professionals should not assume that older adults are less likely to forget to take their medications, unless there is good reason to suppose that they are suffering from memory loss.

Memory loss

Sudden memory loss, confusion and disorientation in older people are commonly due to simple medical conditions, such as respiratory or urinary tract infections, anaemia, or self-neglect associated with malnutrition or dehydration. Treatment usually results in memory restoration unless permanent toxic brain damage has occurred. Memory loss is also a relatively common reaction to a drug or anaesthetic. Correctly assessing the cause of the problem and initiating appropriate treatment should reverse memory loss in most cases. Many older people can remember details of adverse events long afterwards, even though they appeared totally confused at the time. The following scenario illustrates how important it is to explain to people who are in a temporary confused state what is happening:

> Ted's friend Violet, aged 81, described to a researcher what had happened the day after an operation she had had three months previously. She recalled seeing snakes crawling over the lady in the bed opposite and remembered how she kept trying to climb out of bed to remove them. She was aware of becoming more and more agitated as nurses kept dragging her back, until finally one of them explained that these were hallucinations caused by the anaesthetic. She remembered how this explanation calmed her.

Dementias

Alzheimer's disease is probably the best-known form of long-term memory loss and confusion, and is the most common cause of dementia. It is a progressive brain disease that involves loss of memory, confusion, and problems with speech and understanding. The number of people with dementia increases dramatically with age. However, a study by Sliwinski *et al.* (2003) found no direct statistical relationship with chronological age. Instead, they found that progression of pre-clinical dementia was the most important predictor of memory loss. The main risk factor for Alzheimer's disease is genetic. For reasons that are partly genetic but are not yet fully understood, people with learning disabilities are at greater risk of dementia at a much earlier age. Another common type of dementia, vascular dementia, is caused by lifestyle factors such as heavy drinking and smoking, as with other vascular diseases.

Many people remain undiagnosed until the later stages of dementia. This is partly because of difficulties in diagnosis and partly due to the stigma associated with the disease. It is recommended that diagnosis is based on tests of semantic knowledge, verbal recall and simple reasoning abilities (Earnst *et al.* 2000). The test most commonly used to diagnose dementia or Alzheimer's disease is the 'Mini Mental State Examination' (Folstein *et al.* 1975). This requires the individual to name common objects (semantic knowledge), repeat the same objects (verbal recall), and count back from 100 in sevens (reasoning). A test score of less than 24 out of 30 is indicative of dementia. Some authors have drawn attention to the possibility of cultural bias in these types of test, particularly where items involve the use of language or lack cultural relevance (Teresi *et al.* 2001). This means that older members of some immigrant groups are vulnerable to false positive testing using standard measures.

There is no cure for most types of dementia, including Alzheimer's disease. In the early stages, simple memory aids such as writing reminders and making lists can help to overcome forgetfulness. Later, the aim of treatment is not simply to improve memory, but to enable patients and their families to manage and come to terms with the problems of dementia. Depression and anxiety are commonly associated with dementia, but it is difficult to distinguish between cause and effect. Confusion and forgetfulness are likely to increase distress and agitation, while increased anxiety and agitation make the memory problem worse. A number of drug treatments are available. The main psychological treatment is cognitive retraining or stimulation; however, a recent meta-analysis by Clare *et al.* (2003) failed to identify any significant benefits from these.

The caregivers of those with Alzheimer's are particularly at risk of stress-related illness (Chapter 7). Memory problems make reciprocal communication very difficult and take great patience and understanding. It is also tempting to think that once a person's memory has gone, the individual inside has also gone. Many carers experience great distress because the person they love no longer remembers who they are, or may mistake a spouse for a parent or a daughter or son for a deceased wife or husband. People with dementia may ask the same question again and again and never appear to take in the answer. This can become very frustrating and makes the sufferer susceptible to abuse from relatives. It is not easy for professionals either. But aspects of autobiographical memory, particularly those related to emotionally salient events, often remain intact until the very late stages of Alzheimer's disease. Encouraging the person to remember events from their past can be informative as well as rewarding.

Marie Mills (Mills and Walker 1994) conducted in-depth interviews with institutionalized elderly patients who had severe dementia. She encouraged them to talk about their past. She recounted how one particular man, Mr Fellows, initially appeared confused and depressed. Nevertheless, he described detailed episodes from his childhood which his wife, to her surprise, confirmed as accurate. One day he recounted how he had once lost his school cap, which meant his mother had to buy another (they were very poor). The staff confirmed that he would sometimes wander round the ward in an agitated state saying 'where's my cap?'. Later on, Mr Fellows confided how ashamed he was of being incontinent and how annoyed he was that the chiropodist had not attended to his feet. It emerged that he actually had quite a lot of awareness of his current feelings and needs.

As the study progressed, Mr Fellows started to cheer up and became less agitated and depressed. The best explanation for this is that the staff began to respond to him more as an individual with an interesting life history. Mills recommended that a social history should accompany older patients, particularly those needing longer-term care, so that staff are encouraged to treat each person as a unique individual.

In order to save time, autobiographical accounts can be encouraged while engaging in personal care. Alternatively, it may help to involve volunteer 'listeners' to record this information. It does not matter if the events recalled are happy or sad, provided the listener is willing to tolerate the shedding of a few tears. Recalling early memories helps the individual to regain some sense of coherence within their lives (Chapter 2). It also helps care providers to gain a sense of the individual as a person in their own right, rather than just another forgetful old person.

Brain injury

Certain types of brain injury caused by trauma or stroke can lead to particular types of memory loss. We are now venturing into 'abnormal' psychology which as we explained in the Preface, we are unable to cover in depth here. Accidental brain damage may cause complete loss of short-term memory and encoding, such that the individual fails to remember anything that has occurred since the onset of the disorder or trauma. Total memory loss (amnesia) is actually rare. More common are specific types of memory loss associated with damage to different parts of the brain. For example, it is fairly common following cerebral vascular accident (stroke) to find that the individual has unilateral neglect. This means that the patient 'forgets' that they have a left-hand or right-hand side to their body until they are reminded. The arm or leg functions perfectly well when they make a conscious effort to move it, but in the course of trying to walk or feed themselves, they fail to attempt to use it. Some people actually fail to see objects on the left or right. This may be caused by a breakdown in the ability to integrate visual, perceptual and motor information and may respond to a programme of re-education.

Communicating effectively with patients

Volumes have been written about the importance of effective communication. In this chapter, we focus particularly on information-giving and patient understanding. Philip Ley (1997) drew on the principles of memory research to identify a number of ways in which communication between client and health care professional can be improved:

- Improve the environment (avoid delays, be friendly, allow the patient to explain things in their own words).
- Find out what the patient believes and encourage feedback.
- Stress the importance of particular content and repeat it.
- Give important information first and repeat it last.
- Check that you are using language that the patient can understand.
- Give specific, rather than general or vague advice.
- Provide written back-up material, but ensure that this is written and presented so that people can understand it.

Ley (1997) provided a comprehensive research-based analysis of problems of poor communication, much of which is quite old but nevertheless relevant. For example, he explored reasons for taking incorrect medication, including not taking enough, taking too much, incorrect dose interval, incorrect treatment duration and taking additional medications. He found, for example, that patients were often unable to understand quite simple written or verbal instructions. Even instructions such as 'consult your doctor if symptoms persist' were poorly understood by a large number of people. In high school students, words such as 'fatal' and 'misuse' were poorly understood. Among the general public, the words 'infection' and 'cancer' were understood by most people, but the terms 'metastasis' and 'prognosis' were not.

Those preparing to design patient information leaflets would do well to read Ley's book for simple tips on how to improve the chances that patients will read and understand them. This includes using shorter words and shorter sentences. Standard tests of readability may help to ensure this.

But perhaps the most important way of improving written information is to involve representatives of patient or user groups (expert patients) in developing and presenting relevant and appropriate content in a way that is meaningful and accessible to the people who really matter. It is important, whether giving written or verbal information, for practitioners to understand patients' priorities in terms of the information they are likely to wish to receive.

Michie *et al.* (1997) conducted a study of patient knowledge and satisfaction with genetic counselling. Counsellors were asked to indicate important aspects of information given to patients, and this was checked against tape-recordings of the actual consultations. One month later, patients were telephoned and asked to recall as much as they could and to rate its importance. Patients were more likely than counsellors to judge information about family implications as important, while counsellors were more likely to judge information about test, diagnosis and prognosis as important. This indicates that we often do not understand the priorities given by patients to particular aspects of information.

More recent research has examined the effects of bias in information-giving. For example, Hall *et al.* (2003) reported that pregnant women who were given information about the presence of chromosomal abnormalities accompanied by negative statements were far more likely to undergo termination than those who were given information in a neutral or positive way. As a result of their study, the authors recommended that staff adhere to standard protocols for giving sensitive information. Information is very easily biased when given in a negative or apologetic way, and choices manipulated by the ways in which professionals convey information. Compare the following ways in which Sasha might be told that she will have to have her baby in a consultant obstetric unit instead of the midwife-led unit into which she originally booked:

Midwife: Well, Sasha, I'm afraid that we will have to transfer you to the consultant unit.

Midwife: Well, Sasha, we will need to transfer you to our friends over in the consultant unit.

Subtle differences in the ways that information is conveyed can make a lot of difference to the way that it is perceived. For Sasha, it could make the difference between acceptance and fear.

Breaking bad news

The analysis of Lillian's experience of being told about having cancer high-lights just how difficult it is for people to remember information when being given bad news about their diagnosis. Lesley Fallowfield was the first psychologist to study the effects of offering patients a tape recording of the 'bad news' consultation (Hogbin and Fallowfield 1989) so that patients could listen again at their leisure. This does not suit everybody, but those who have elected to do this have found it extremely helpful in gaining a better understanding of the whole situation, and in explaining it to close family or friends. Fallowfield has since investigated other aspects of the bad news consultation.

Fallowfield and her co-researchers observed that health care professionals often censor information in an attempt to protect patients from potentially distressing information. However, she argued that the well-intentioned desire to shield patients from the reality of their situation usually creates even greater difficulties for patients, caregivers and members of the health care team, since it leads to a conspiracy of silence and heightened state of anxiety and confusion. 'Ambiguous or deliberately misleading information may afford short-term benefits while things continue to go well, but denies individuals and their families opportunities to reorganize and adapt their lives towards the attainment of more achievable goals, realistic hopes and aspirations' (Fallowfield *et al.* 2002: 297).

Michelle Crossley (2003) used John Diamond's personal account of oral cancer to illustrate problems faced by cancer patients. For example, Diamond described how when he told others he had cancer, they heard him say that he was about to die. For many people, the cancer schema implies death. But Crossley drew on Diamond's own words to describe how, when offered the possibility of treatment, patients tend to cling on to 'an almost childish belief in the power of modern medicine'. Those working in the field of cancer and palliative care have a natural wish to sustain hope, but tread a fine line between what is realistic and what is unrealistic.

A good way to establish people's needs and wishes for information is to undertake some 'what if' explorations at an early stage.

When Lillian originally went for her biopsy, her doctor explained that the results would show whether or not she had cancer. The doctor asked her how she might feel if she did have cancer, and what sort of information she would wish to be told. When the results came through, the doctor reminded Lillian of what she had said and asked her if she had changed her mind. She was then given the sort of information that she was best able to cope with.

Walker (1989) asked older people 'if you had something seriously wrong with you, would you like to know all about it, even if the outlook was not good?'. Eighty per cent said that they would wish to know, indicating that you can only deal with what you know about. Ten per cent were unconcerned, and only 10% said that they would not wish to know, so that they could keep their dreams and hopes. Some commented that they might not have been so keen to know when they were younger.

Forgetting bad news

A number of explanations for forgetting bad news have already been given. Freud argued that painful memories are repressed, or forced out of the conscious mind. Repression is one of several defence mechanisms that defend the ego, or sense of self, against harsh external realities. Denial is another. Denial refers to the failure of people to acknowledge the reality of a situation that causes great anxiety. This may offer protection in the short term, since the individual does not have to face up to the difficult realities. Some argue that denial is an effective coping mechanism when death is imminent, as in a terminal illness. But it can lead to problems of communication between patient, caregivers and professionals, as observed by Fallowfield *et al.* (2002).

Individualized information-giving

It is difficult to judge the amount and type of information that an individual person wants or needs. The best approach, as illustrated above, is to elicit what the patient already understands, find out what they wish to know, and check afterwards what they have understood. When faced with the possibility of having to give bad news, it is preferable to negotiate information needs with the patient before investigations are carried out and results received. At that point, it is possible to find out whether or not people want to know every detail of the causes and likely consequences of their illness. This seems rarely to be done in practice, and not doing it can lead to unfortunate consequences. It is not uncommon for relatives to try to protect their loved ones by requesting that they should not be given bad news. This is not only unethical, but can in many instances interfere with communication. Good practice in information-giving starts and ends with listening.

Summary of key points

- The ability to remember verbal information is poor but can be enhanced by reducing the amount of information given, taking care with the order in which it is given and emphasizing key issues.
- People are unlikely to remember information that does not fit with their existing framework of understanding (schema). Therefore, it is important to take time to find out a patient's current understanding and then to build on it.
- When dealing with patients with severe memory loss, taking the time to explain what is happening can reduce anxiety and agitation.
- People's need for information varies, and it is helpful to find out what and how much people want to know when embarking on a course of investigation or treatment.
- Listening to individual needs and respecting individual wishes are essential components of care.

Further reading

Ley, P. (1997) *Communicating with Patients: Improving Satisfaction and Compliance*. Cheltenham: Stanley Thornes.

CHAPTER FOUR

LEARNING AND SOCIAL LEARNING

- How can we learn to respond without being aware of it?
- What influences the way we learn to respond to different situations?
- How can we apply learning theory to treat fears, anxieties and phobias?
- How can behavioural and social learning theories inform us about factors that need to be taken into account when encouraging lifestyle change?
- What is 'learned helplessness' and how does this account for depression?
- How can we use learning theories to help manage our own lives and improve the lives of others?

Introduction

This chapter focuses on theories of learning developed from behavioural psychology. These theories direct attention to situational causes of behaviour that are amenable to change. Behavioural theories can be helpful in understanding how a range of health-related behaviours and emotional responses are acquired, influenced and maintained, and how they can be managed or treated. These theories have been used to develop evidence-based approaches to behaviour management and change in a variety of clinical settings during the past few decades.

We describe aspects of behavioural and social learning theory that are relevant to health and health care. We seek to demonstrate how they can be used to explain and change some common health-related behaviours. We consider the contribution of these theories to the development of cognitive behavioural treatment programmes.

Types of learning

It is tempting to confuse learning with memory because much educational learning seems to involve memorizing. However, a lot of learning does not involve deliberate activity – for example, learning how to make relationships, learning new skills, learning how and when to avoid difficult situations, learning how to behave in different social settings, and learning how to ride a bike. Some of these behaviours might be described as innate, some involve trial and error, some involve watching and copying others, some can be learned from books or manuals or are taught by others, but a surprising amount of learning takes place without our even being aware of it.

In this chapter, we focus on conditioning theories and social learning theory because these have particular relevance to health and health care. 'Learning theory' in academic psychology refers specifically to theories developed by behaviourists or behavioural psychologists. Behaviourists were the first psychologists to engage in the systematic study of learning processes, based mainly on animal experiments. They used behaviour change as evidence that learning had taken place and did not concern themselves with mental processes. However, more recent experiments have made it possible for psychologists to draw inferences about beliefs associated with behaviour change. This has enabled behavioural learning principles to be incorporated into cognitive science and cognitive behavioural therapies.

Background to the development of learning theory

It is helpful to have some insight into the thinking behind conditioning theory. Philosophers and psychologists have tended to subscribe to one of two views about the nature of human learning: **nativism** and **empiricism**. Nativists believe that humans have a unique set of innate abilities that enable them to acquire and organize knowledge in a special way. Language is cited as a good example of this because children learn very quickly how to apply rules of grammar. In contrast, empiricists believe that we are born *tabula rasa* (literally 'blank slate') and that all knowledge is gained from experience. Empiricists prior to the twentieth century believed that learning took place by association. Association might be because objects or situations look similar to each other in some way; or because events occur together at the same time; or because one event always precedes another, implying a relationship of cause and effect. Behaviourism grew out of empiricism.

Behaviourists, with encouragement from Darwin's theory of evolution, made no distinction between the learning processes of animals and humans, and claimed that theories derived from animal studies could be applied to human beings. They also claimed that the only legitimate way to demonstrate learning was to observe the ways living organisms respond to external stimuli. This attracted the name 'stimulus-response theory'. Behaviourists did not deny the existence of thought processes but claimed that these are 'private events' that cannot be studied objectively. More recently, however, conditioning theories have been reinterpreted in terms of the underlying set of beliefs or expectations. This has enabled behavioural learning principles to be incorporated into cognitive psychology and, more recently, cognitive science. These principles form important components of cognitive behavioural therapies.

Conditioning theories

Conditioning refers to simple forms of associative learning. Two types of conditioning were identified during the last century, classical conditioning and operant conditioning. Classical conditioning involves reflex responses (those over which we nave no conscious control). Operant conditioning involves voluntary responses (those over which we normally have conscious control).

Classical conditioning

Classical conditioning is the simplest form of associative learning. Ivan Pavlov first recorded the phenomenon of classical conditioning during studies of the digestive systems of dogs. Dogs, like humans, salivate when they see food; it is a natural physiological reflex response. But Pavlov demonstrated that a signal, such as a bell, if presented immediately before giving the dog food, would eventually lead the dog to salivate to the sound of the bell. Salivation to a bell is a 'conditioned' or learned response.

This type of learning has clear implications for health and health care. A typical illustration involves the child who is afraid of the doctor (Figure 4.1).

When he went for immunization at 15 months old, Lee was quite happy to see the doctor. Then the doctor gave Lee his immunization, which hurt a lot. Lee now associates the doctor with pain and howls with protest at his approach to the doctor's surgery

Lee learned from his experience that going to see the doctor predicts the possibility of having an injection that causes a lot of pain. Therefore he cries and protests whenever he approaches the surgery.

Prevention is always better than cure. One way to reduce the impact of an injection for the pre-verbal child is to distract their attention while they have the injection, and reward them immediately afterwards with a treat. Hopefully, they will then come to associate the doctor with something pleasant, rather than the painful injection.

Adults, too, are susceptible to conditioned responses in health care settings.

Lillian felt very sick as a result of her first chemotherapy treatment. As she approached the hospital for her second treatment, she started to feel sick again.

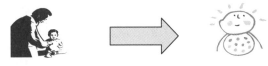

The child is happy in the presence of the doctor

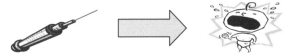

The doctor gives the child an injection that hurts

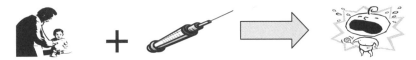

The child now associates the doctor with the painful injection

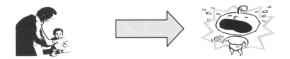

So the child screams when the doctor appears

Figure 4.1 Classically conditioned fear of the doctor.

Many patients undergoing chemotherapy feel nauseous at the sight or smell of the hospital. This is a classically conditioned response. It is difficult to gain conscious control over this type of reaction once it has become a conditioned response. Therefore, it is important to prevent the development of the conditioned response by giving the patient an anti-emetic drug following their first chemotherapy to inhibit nausea.

Another example of classical conditioning is the triggering of an asthmatic attack. Asthma is caused by the constriction of the bronchus in response to an allergen. So how is it that someone who is allergic to the fur of a cat or dog may find that their asthmatic attack is triggered by the sight of a cat or dog in the distance, or even by a picture of a cat or dog? It used to be believed that this type of response indicated that asthma was a **psychogenic** disorder (all in the mind). But medical research has since shown conclusively that asthma is caused by an allergic response. The best explanation is that classical conditioning has taken place.

For years, Jo believed that his symptoms of hay fever were caused by allergy to cats. He experienced itchy eyes and runny nose whenever a cat

entered the room. More recently, he discovered from skin tests that he is actually allergic to house dust mite and not cats. House dust mite cells are present in bedding and allergic responses are often worse on waking. The appearance of the cat first thing in the morning was probably sufficient to generate an association between the cat and the hay fever symptoms.

Other reflexes amenable to classical conditioning include anxiety, fear or panic, urinary and anal sphincter control, hunger, thirst, sexual arousal, facial ticks and other body movements or mannerisms.

The principles of classical conditioning have led to the development of a number of important and widely used interventions, an example of which is the pad and bell used to stop bed wetting in older children. The child sleeps soundly and fails to recognize or respond to the urge to urinate. Sensitive pads are placed under the sheet and wired to a bell. The bell sounds as soon as urine touches the pads and wakes the child up to get out of bed and use the toilet. The bell prompts the association of urination with waking. Over a period of time, the urge to urinate wakes the child in time to get to the toilet.

There are two important points to remember when applying the principle of classical conditioning. First, a conditioned response is not under conscious or voluntary control. For example, asthma sufferers are quite unable to use will power to stop themselves having an attack in response to a picture of a cat. Second, all autonomic responses (those involving the arousal of the sympathetic and parasympathetic nervous systems) are capable of this type of conditioning. This includes emotional responses such as anxiety and fear.

Conditioned emotional responses

An emotion consists of:

- a belief (about what is happening);
- a set of behavioural responses (such as smiling or crying);
- a state of autonomic arousal (stimulation of the autonomic nervous system).

Autonomic responses, and hence emotions, are very susceptible to classical conditioning. This offers a simple explanation for many fears and phobias. Classical conditioning theory has been shown experimentally to explain fear responses.

Watson and Rayner demonstrated in 1920 how an 11-month-old child named Albert, who had shown no previous fear, was conditioned to be frightened of a white rat. This followed a period in which the rat was held in front of the child at the same time as a loud banging on his cot. The banging aroused strong fear and the rat became associated with the fear response. More important, Albert subsequently showed a fear of anything that was white and furry. The transfer of the conditioned fear response from one object to other similar objects is called 'generalization'.

Most associations take repeated experiences to develop. However, exposure to a single intense stimulus that leads to a strong autonomic fear response can sometimes be enough to cause a conditioned fear response. For example, someone who has been in a very frightening road or rail accident may be too scared to get into any type of moving transport after that, even though they are well aware that the chances of it happening again are extremely rare. This may be a contributory cause of post-traumatic stress disorder (PTSD). Equally, fears associated with illness, hospitals or medical procedures may come about as a result of a single frightening or painful event. PTSD has been identified following myocardial infarction, childbirth and intensive care treatment as well as a number of other experiences (Tedstone and Tarrier 2003). Tedstone and Tarrier identified the main cause as poor support and negative interactions with health care staff. This appears to highlight the importance of good therapeutic management practices to reduce anxiety and fear.

The importance of fear reduction in hospital settings

Classically conditioned fear or anxiety responses are troublesome and difficult to treat. Therefore prevention is always better than cure. In hospital settings, this can be achieved through better patient preparation for planned procedures. For example, nurses, doctors and therapists can help patients to anticipate potentially frightening or painful stimuli (injections, procedures, etc.) so that they do not experience sudden or unexpected fear, pain or other unpleasant experiences. It is often claimed that it is not necessary to concern patients with potential negative experiences, since this could lead to a self-fulfilling prophecy. There is no evidence to support this belief and plenty of evidence to the contrary. Most people who are well prepared for and supported during a procedure do not experience such a high level of arousal. They are able to recognize and understand what is happening and know how to respond appropriately.

Lee needed to go to hospital for a planned procedure. The staff on the unit recognized the importance of preparing Lee for this. They had a pre-operation clinic where Lee could see the surroundings, meet other children, and watch a video showing what procedures he would experience. Staff encouraged Lee to rehearse these with a doll. This reduced the likelihood of a conditioned fear response and also reduced Sasha's anxieties about Lee's operation.

Reasonable or rational argument is not effective for someone whose fear response has already been conditioned. In fact, fears, anxieties and phobias acquired in this way are often described as 'irrational' because the individual has no logical reason to be frightened.

Fear and avoidance

One way some individuals deal with situations that cause fear or anxiety is to avoid them. For example, many people avoid going for dental checks because of their fear of the dentist. However, conditioned responses remain strong in the absence of the stimulus that triggers them, and avoidance can lead to a phobia. As a result, some people prefer to risk having a general anaesthetic for tooth extraction than have it done at the dentist under safer local anaesthetic.

Many phobias appear to involve fear of fear, rather than fear of a particular consequence. In extreme situations, avoidance can lead to crippling restrictions on lifestyle and quality of life.

Crombez et al. (1999) noted that pain-related fear is more disabling than the pain itself. Acute pain alerts us to tissue damage and requires immediate action. Escape and avoidance are adaptive responses to accidental pain, since they remove us from the cause and ensure that we avoid future exposure to a dangerous situation. Many chronic pains have persisted after healing has taken place. But people with chronic pain equate pain with harm and try to avoid movements that they believe cause pain. Therefore they avoid exercise, work and many everyday tasks because they fear further damage.

Phobias are persistent fears of specific objects or situations. For example, agoraphobia refers to a fear of open spaces. In many cases, the individual has experienced a panic attack (sudden intense arousal of the autonomic nervous system) while in a public place and is afraid of this happening again. It leads people to avoid going out of the house and can have serious social consequences.

The best-known therapeutic approach to the treatment of fears and phobias, based on the principles of classical conditioning, was developed by Joseph Wolpe (1958) and is called systematic desensitization.

Systematic desensitization

Anxiety and fear involve autonomic responses that cause breathing, pulse rate and blood pressure to increase and muscles to tense. The patient is therefore taught techniques that oppose these responses. They learn to relax all major muscles and controlled breathing techniques. Then they learn to apply the relaxation technique in a 'hierarchical' series of situations that are graded in terms of threat. For example, first they might be asked to imagine a mild fear-producing situation while practising relaxation. Once they can achieve this without fear, they imagine more severe fear-producing situations. They might progress to looking at pictures or films, then to thinking about approaching the actual situation, and finally to exposure to the feared situation in the company of the therapist. The precise programme will vary according to the nature and severity of the problem. At each stage, the individual must demonstrate complete control through relaxation before proceeding to the next stage.

Systematic desensitization has a long history of successfully treating a wide variety of incapacitating and long-standing conditioned fear and anxiety responses. Further, Wolpe recognized that many fears and phobias occur in response to social demands or situations. Therefore, he recommended assertiveness training as an additional means of helping people to gain control over anxiety-provoking social encounters. This means training them to stand up for themselves and their needs in a non-confrontational way. It remains an important component of cognitive behavioural therapy treatments.

Operant (instrumental) conditioning

Operant or instrumental conditioning refers to the learned association between voluntary actions and their consequences or outcomes. Operant conditioning applies to voluntary behaviours – those over which we normally have conscious control.

Operant conditioning theory proposes that learning takes place as a result of reinforcement and punishment. For example, I learn from experience that eating strawberries is pleasurable, so I eat more. In this case, the strawberry is termed a 'reinforcer' because it increases the likelihood that my behaviour (eating them) will be repeated. Alternatively, I learn that if I touch a hot iron I will burn myself so I do not touch it again. Here the hot iron is termed a 'punisher' because it decreases the likelihood that I will repeat the action.

The terms **reinforcement** and **punishment** have particular meaning for behaviourists, for whom reinforcement does not necessarily mean the same as reward.

When the new baby was born, Lee became more naughty. Sasha scolded him, believing that this was a punishment. However, Lee viewed the scold as attention and repeated the naughty behaviour to gain more of his mother's attention. Therefore, in behaviourist terms, the scold is defined as a reinforcer.

A 'primary reinforcer' is something that fulfils basic needs, such as food, drink or sex. Substances such as nicotine and crack cocaine may also be regarded as primary reinforcers because they satisfy physiological needs. A 'secondary reinforcer' is one that provides a source of primary reinforcement. Receiving help from other people may be regarded as a form of secondary reinforcement, and some illness behaviours are described as achieving secondary gain, because they enable the patient to avoid difficult or painful tasks.

The psychologist famous for the development of the principles of operant conditioning was B.F. Skinner. Operant principles were derived from animal laboratory experiments and used such equipment as the 'Skinner box'. This was a cage in which a light or sound was used to signal to the animal or bird that, if it pressed a lever or pecked a key, it would receive a food reward. Thus animals were trained to respond to different types of stimulus or cue, and the effect on the animal's behaviour of different patterns or schedules of reinforcement was measured. Below, we have illustrated some operant concepts and principles that are useful in practice.

Context and cues

Individuals quickly learn that particular actions have certain consequences only in specific situations or contexts that act as cues.

Sasha scolded Lee when he attempted to go near the fire. This stopped him from approaching the fire in her presence, so she assumed that it was now safe to leave him alone in the room when the fire was lit. However, as soon as Sasha left the room, Lee attempted to poke the fire. He had learned not to touch the fire, but only in the presence of his mother.

Many health-related behaviours are described as under **stimulus control**. That is to say, they are automatic responses to environmental cues.

> Jo lights up a cigarette automatically as soon as he sits down to drink a cup of coffee. Lighting up a cigarette is normally considered to be a conscious or voluntary response, but becomes automatic in certain situations. Similarly, someone may get into the habit of pouring a drink when they arrive home from work.

An important reason why **health-related behaviours**, such as smoking, fail to respond to health promotion or health education is that in many situations they are not the product of conscious thought. Rather they are habits that involve automatic responses to particular environmental or internal cues. Once someone has expressed the desire to give up smoking, it is necessary to interrupt these habitual routines and bring the behaviour back under conscious control.

Schedules of reinforcement or punishment

The term 'schedule' refers to a sequential pattern of reinforcement or punishment. For example, it may be continuous (happen every time) or intermittent (happen only occasionally). Sometimes an occasional intense reward or punishment can influence behaviour more strongly than continuous but less intense ones. Gambling is a good example of how one large win (or even the possibility of one) can provide strong motivation to continue for a very long time. The intense effects of crack cocaine may help to explain the speed of addiction. Similarly, one intense unpleasant experience may act as a deterrent (as in the principle of the short, sharp shock).

Continuous reinforcement may lead to satiation. For example, if we always praise people or seek to reassure people, this is eventually taken for granted and ceases to enhance their performance. Certain drugs such as opioid analgesics, if taken regularly over a long period of time, also seem to have a reduced effect. Therefore, people with chronic pain gradually have to increase the dose in order to achieve the same effect.

The subjective nature of reinforcement and punishment

Reinforcement is not necessarily the same thing as reward. Food is only reinforcing if someone is hungry and likes the food on offer. The child who receives little adult attention may behave badly to provoke punishment as a source of attention. Therefore one person's punishment is another person's reward. Smoking is a good illustration of this. Smoking may seem a disgusting habit to a non-smoker, but it has a number of highly reinforcing consequences for the smoker, including:

- pleasure or satisfaction;
- relaxation or stress management;

- maintaining alertness;
- social bonding;
- time out from demanding or difficult situations;
- having something to do with the hands.

In order to help the smoker give up smoking, it is necessary to explore all the reinforcing effects of smoking. Then it is necessary to plan how to substitute for the effects of each of these. You will note that only the first three of these benefits are a direct consequence of nicotine. Therefore, nicotine patches or chewing gum are only part of the solution.

Hilary Graham (1993) conducted a qualitative research study to find out why working-class women smoked when they could ill afford to. She found that smoking provided 'time out' from their dreary and demanding lives. One woman explained that when she lit her cigarette, it was a cue for the children to leave her alone. The cigarette provided her with personal time and space.

The immediacy of the consequence

Generally, the more immediate the consequence of an action, the more powerful its effect. Small children will normally choose to have a small chocolate bar now, rather than wait for a large one later (assuming they like chocolate). As we grow older, we learn to delay gratification, but the effect of an immediate reward is still powerful.

Consider the list of reasons why smokers smoke. You may notice that the consequences are all immediate. On the other hand, the adverse consequences of smoking on health may be many years hence. This may be an important reason why smokers are not persuaded to give up smoking for health reasons, unless or until they experience symptoms of illness (Walker 1993).

Punishment frequently fails to work because it is administered long after the crime was committed. Chastising a child when the misdemeanour is discovered, rather than when it was committed, is unlikely to have the desired effect unless accompanied by a clear explanation of what they have done wrong. In the absence of the explanation, the child is likely to interpret the displeasure as directed at them, meaning 'I am a bad person', rather than realizing that the punishment is directed at their behaviour.

It appears that some consequences are not affected by delay. For example, experiments have shown that rats made ill by poison will subsequently avoid the type of food or drink that contained the poison, even though there is a substantial delay between eating the food and being ill (Garcia *et al.* 1966). This type of association clearly has survival value and has given rise to the argument that some responses are innately primed or prepared.

The certainty of the consequences

In order to have any impact on behaviour, the reinforcing or punishing consequences must be either certain or very likely to occur. An important reason why punishment fails to eliminate or reduce crime is that the chances of getting caught are not great. The same applies to the perceived chances of getting ill.

> Janice tried to persuade Jo to cut down on his smoking and drinking for health reasons. But the reinforcing consequences of cigarettes and alcohol were all predictable and certain. In contrast, Jo could see no certainty that he was likely to get ill as a result or smoking or drinking. He cited the example of his uncle who smoked and drank heavily but lived to a ripe old age.

This leads to the conclusion that healthy people are less likely to take preventative health advice because they have never been ill and therefore do not associate their behaviour with illness. Many people fail to take action until symptoms occur, and this may be too late. The perceived likelihood of getting ill becomes greater as one grows older. This may be a reason why more people attempt to change their lifestyles later in life.

Lifestyle and behaviour

Behaviours such as smoking, eating, drinking and exercise play important roles in filling time in our lives. Therefore if someone wishes to give up one behaviour, it is necessary to replace it with something else which is equally rewarding and occupies similar space in their lives. This means that the reinforcing consequences of smoking, drinking or drug-taking need to be replaced with equally desirable alternatives if a programme of lifestyle change is to be effective (DiClemente 1993).

> Jo enjoys drinking seven or eight pints of beer with his mates at the pub. This is not because he is thirsty, but because it is a relaxing social activity that makes for a pleasant evening out. Sasha wants him to cut down on his drinking. But if he wants to spend the same time with his mates, he will need to find an alternative that provides similar sources of reinforcement. A low-alcohol lager may seem a reasonable alternative, but is more expensive, does not taste the same, and does not have the social approval of his drinking companions. It is very difficult to address individual behaviour in binge-drinking culture.

Taking up a new health-related behaviour such as exercise requires extra time and space within an individual's lifestyle, therefore another activity will need to be displaced. If exercise is to be maintained, it must be more reinforcing for the individual than alternative ways of using their time. Try applying this principle to dieting. You will soon see that it is easier to diet if foods that increase weight are exchanged for similar quantities of food that are just as desirable but do not put on weight. Perhaps this helps to explain the success of the Atkins diet?

Behaviour modification

Behaviour modification means changing behaviour by deliberately manipulating its context and/or reinforcement and is based directly upon the operant principles of B.F. Skinner. During the 1970s, behaviour modification became a popular way to control socially undesirable or obsessive behaviours in long-stay mental health institutions, using a token economy. This meant that socially desirable behaviours were reinforced by immediately giving tokens that could be exchanged for primary reinforcers of the patient's choice (sadly, this often took the form of cigarettes). Antisocial behaviour was ignored, not punished. Punishment had no place in Skinner's approach to behaviour modification. There are many simple forms of behaviour modification still in common use. For example, principles of classroom management include giving attention for good behaviour and ignoring bad behaviour.

Behaviour modification is often used to cure bed-wetting once a child is capable of achieving bladder control. This involves using a 'star chart'. Every dry morning, a star is placed by the child on a specially prepared chart. Once an agreed number of stars has been acquired, these can be exchanged for a present of the child's choice. The child is never chastized for having a wet bed, only rewarded for a dry one. Similar approaches can be used to eliminate temper tantrums or other challenging behaviours, provided the child is able to understand the process (Chapter 5).

Behaviour modification does not always work as intended.

Janice's friend had a child who was reluctant to eat, so his parents started rewarding him with money each time he finished a meal. The child eventually had enough money to buy his own television set. But by that time he refused to eat at all unless he was paid.

Before embarking on a programme of behaviour modification, it is necessary to consider the possibility of any unintended or adverse consequences.

Functional analysis of behaviour

Functional analysis of behaviour is an important part of behaviour modification and involves monitoring the ABC (antecedents, behaviour and consequences) of behaviour. Behaviourists recommend that before any programme of behaviour change is started, the frequency of the problem behaviour should be recorded in a diary, together with the immediate causes (antecedents) and immediate consequences (sources of reinforcement). This process can be applied to someone planning to give up smoking, or to a parent who wishes to eliminate their child's temper tantrums, or to someone who wishes to improve their timekeeping. The process and the principles are illustrated in relation to Lee's tantrums:

> *Baseline measures.* Sasha recorded how often the tantrums occurred during the course of a week.
> *Identify stimulus cues.* In addition to recording the number of tantrums, Sasha recorded what was happening at the time each tantrum started. This enabled her to develop strategies to distract Lee from situations likely to cause tantrums.
> *Identify reinforcers or punishers.* Sasha also recorded what happened as a result of Lee's tantrums. For example, did he stop as soon as she gave him what he was demanding?
>
> Having collected this information, Sasha then introduced a system of 'time out' (removing him from the scene), or ignoring him, when he was having a tantrum, and giving him more attention at other times.
>
> *Measurement of change.* She continued to monitor the frequency of Lee's tantrums to provide feedback on progress.

Over a period of three weeks, Lee's tantrums reduced dramatically. By this time, Sasha felt much more confident in dealing with his behaviour. She identified that most tantrums occurred when she was trying to do some housework, and this enabled her to prepare diversionary activities. The extra attention at other times also seemed to help.

Self-modification

The principles of applied behaviour analysis can be used to help us change all sorts of aspects of our own behaviour, for example, being late for work or being short-tempered with our partner or spouse. This involves the following steps:

1. Decide which aspect of behaviour needs to change.
2. Monitor the frequency, causes and consequences of the behaviour.

3. Study the pattern of behaviour and identify persistent cues or consequences.
4. Plan to alter routines or respond differently to stimulus cues.
5. Substitute reinforcers for undesired behaviour with rewards or treats for desired behaviour.
6. Measure the change in frequency of occurrence.
7. Maintain change with treats or self-praise to reinforce successful behaviour and boost self-esteem. Quite often the improvement is sufficient to maintain the change, but treats act as a reminder.

> Anna was finding it difficult to get out of bed in the mornings. She was missing lectures and on two occasions arrived late. She needed to address this urgently. She decided to get in some special treats for breakfast to tempt herself out of bed.

Illness behaviours

The term **illness behaviour** was introduced by Mechanic in the early 1960s to describe the different ways that people perceive, evaluate and act on their illness, much of which is determined by what is culturally acceptable. For example, it is well documented that people in different cultures express pain differently, from the British stiff upper lip to the more expressive responses of the Jewish and Hispanic peoples (Zborowski 1969).

Illness behaviours include engaging in self-care activities, seeking help, advice and reassurance, and doing nothing and ignoring the problem. But the term is more often used to describe abnormal or **maladaptive** ways of responding. Therefore, much of the research into this concept seeks to describe how the behaviour of the patient deviates from that which appears to be justified by the extent of their illness. For example, if medical help-seeking seems excessive, the patient may be stigmatized as a hypochondriac or malingerer (see Chapter 2). People with conditions that are difficult to diagnose, such as chronic back pain, are particularly at risk of these assumptions.

Illness behaviour is more likely to occur in those who are anxious (Rief *et al.* 2003). This is probably because uncertainty about the nature or consequences of an illness prompts the individual to persist in seeking help until they find an answer (Chapter 8). There appear to be cultural differences in the level and duration of symptoms that people from different countries expect to experience, and this, too, will have an effect on help-seeking behaviour (de Melker *et al.* 1997).

There are also behavioural explanations for illness behaviours. Many are behaviours that have been reinforced by the responses of others. Chronic pain is a useful example of this. Craig (2004) described how pain produces expressive behaviours, such as crying, wincing and other non-verbal expressions of pain and distress. These attract the attention of others who recognize suffering and respond by offering help and protection.

> Flor *et al.* (1987) investigated the role of patients' significant others as primary reinforcers in the maintenance of pain behaviours and found that, particularly in married male patients, the attentive responses of spouses led to a significant increase in reports of pain.

It is natural to want to help someone you love and to protect them from pain. But if a caregiver responds by taking over the recipient's former tasks or roles, the person in pain gradually becomes less active and more dependent, pain behaviours become more exaggerated, and the pain gradually becomes chronic.

Fordyce (1982) developed behavioural treatments to reduce pain behaviours and increase activity levels in people with chronic pain. His programme required caregivers to recognize and ignore pain behaviours, while giving encouragement for any kind of activity. This seems quite harsh, but some of these principles have been incorporated into cognitive behavioural therapies for chronic pain, in which patients and caregivers learn to recognize the negative consequences of responding in an attentive way to pain behaviours and change their responses through a process of self-modification. It is termed 'cognitive behavioural' because the programme aims to make the patient fully aware of the principles underlying this approach to therapy, so that they can become actively engaged in changing behaviours that are maladaptive.

Reinforcement or control?

For years, behaviourists focused experiments on the effects of positive or negative consequences in the belief that these were responsible for behaviour. It therefore came as something of a surprise when researchers discovered situations in which the effect was clearly not due to this. Rather, behaviour maintenance and behaviour change were found to be a consequence of the degree of control the animal or human had over positive or negative outcomes. This fitted with the idea that one of the key motivators of human behaviour is to gain mastery over our environment. This line of inquiry had clear implications for health care. For example, it led to a series of studies of the beneficial effects of pre-operative information-giving on the premise that this enhances sense of control and reduces anxiety.

Experiments conducted during the 1960s and 1970s led to a large body of research into the concept of control. Experimental evidence accumulated to show that humans are able to tolerate higher levels of discomfort if they believe they have some means of controlling it. This explains why, for example, we enjoy the fresh air when we open the window ourselves, but complain about the draught when someone else does so! It is also the principle underlying patient-controlled analgesia.

Bowers (1968) conducted an experiment into the relationship between pain tolerance and control. He administered electric shocks to volunteers (university students) who were randomly allocated to one of two groups. Each group was told that the shocks would gradually increase in intensity. One group was told that they could terminate the shock at the press of a button. The other group was advised that they could terminate the experiment by leaving the room. Both groups were advised to continue for as long as they could. Bowers found that those who had an immediate means of personal control by pressing the button tolerated much higher levels of shock than those in the other group. These findings led eventually to the introduction of patient-controlled analgesia.

A similar principle applies to the use of transcutaneous electrical nerve stimulation (TENS) for the management of pain. TENS involves placing small adhesive conductive pads near to the site of the pain, leading to a small control box that releases a small controllable amount of electric current. The electric current stimulates the large pain fibres and overrides the pain signals. It has been shown to be effective in the relief of certain types of pain, including arthritic knee pain (Osiri *et al.* 2003). It has the added advantage in that it is self-operated by the patient and provides a sense of personal control over the pain. This explains why many people report it to be beneficial even if there is no noticeable reduction in pain intensity.

As control emerged as an important concept in psychology, psychologists were also investigating the effects of uncontrollability.

Learned helplessness, uncontrollability and depression

For many years it had been noted that some experimental animals showed symptoms of what was termed 'experimental neurosis'. Basically, they cowered in a corner and could not be persuaded to participate in further experiments. Seligman and Maier (1967) demonstrated that this behaviour was caused by uncontrollability.

Two dogs were administered a series of identical minor electric shocks. One dog (the executive dog) was able to terminate the shock by pressing a panel with its muzzle. This terminated the shock delivered to itself and the other dog, so that both dogs received exactly the same intensity and duration of shock. The only difference was that one dog had control over the shock, while the other had none.

The dogs were then transferred to another experimental environment called a shuttle box. Each dog was placed at one end of a metal box and a minor electric shock delivered through the floor. Both dogs could easily escape by jumping over a low hurdle to safety. In this situation, the executive dog quickly learned to jump over the hurdle to avoid the shock. In contrast, the other dog made no attempt to escape. The 'helpless' dog demonstrated a motivational deficit (it made no attempt to move), a cognitive deficit (it failed to recognize a simple escape route), and an emotional deficit (it appeared very miserable). Seligman termed this 'learned helplessness'.

According to Seligman, learned helplessness means learning that one's actions have no influence on outcomes. It therefore means perceived uncontrollability. Seligman (1975) noted that these motivational, cognitive and emotional deficits are all symptomatic of human depression and proposed learned helplessness as a theory of human depression. The theory of learned helplessness predicts that people become depressed because of exposure to situations or events that they are unable to control. Subsequent researchers have applied this in different types of situations, including social settings.

Lack of control over important aspects of life has been suggested as a reason for the higher incidence of depression among the unemployed, those on low pay, those with less education, and women. Mirowsky and Ross (2003) argue that depression among these groups is caused by their powerlessness in society and not by personal depressive tendencies that have brought them down the social scale.

Learned helplessness has much intuitive appeal. It highlights the dangers of depriving people of control, focuses on external causes of depression, and implies that what has been learned can be unlearned. In contrast, cognitive theories of depression emphasize the importance of pessimistic belief sets that lead people to feel they have little control. These points of view are in fact complementary since what really matters is *perceived* control, not actual control.

Mark started feeling quite depressed after he retired from work due to ill health. He had experienced one previous bout of depression, which had lifted when he changed his job (Chapter 7). Now, he felt that he had lost control over his life and felt helpless. Other people envied his freedom to do other things, but he could not be bothered. He demonstrated the

> motivational, cognitive and emotional deficits typical of learned
> helplessness: he made no effort to do anything, did not believe that he
> was capable of achieving anything more in his life, and felt depressed.

Since the 1970s, learned helplessness has been subject to a number of critiques and reformulations (using **attribution theory**) and ultimately challenged by the academic community as a theory of depression. Nevertheless, there is still powerful evidence from social psychology and **psychoneuroimmunology** to support the relationship between uncontrollability, depression and health outcomes (Chapter 7).

Undoing learned helplessness

Seligman and his colleagues (Seligman *et al.* 1968) experimented with helpless dogs and found that they could be cured if the experimenter physically dragged them across the barrier on numerous occasions to demonstrate that it was possible to escape from the shock. This observation was used to develop behavioural interventions for depression.

> Mark was referred to a clinical psychologist who invited him to review his
> skills and identify some achievable goals that would motivate him and
> restore his sense of control. Mark focused on cooking. Janice worked with
> him to identify suitable recipes and ingredients, and soon Mark was
> preparing some lovely healthy meals. Success breeds success, and Mark's
> depression decreased as he started to regain control over some aspects of
> his life and feel useful, rather than helpless.

The concept of control has enabled learning theory to be integrated into cognitive science, where terms such as reinforcement are no longer used. Control has also replaced the concept of reinforcement in the context of therapy.

Social learning theory

The behavioural experiments and treatments so far described are very much focused on the individual. But humans are social beings who live in complex social contexts. It might therefore seem obvious that the majority of human learning takes place in a social environment, but most early behavioural experiments failed to take account of this. Social learning theory emerged in response to this criticism in the 1960s.

There are two important strands to social learning theory. One is usually attributed to Rotter (1966) and concerns the concept of **locus of control**. The other is attributable to Albert Bandura and focuses on the concepts of observational learning and self-efficacy. More recently, these two strands have been brought together under the heading of **social cognition**.

Observational learning

Albert Bandura is one of the great original thinkers in behavioural psychology. He emerged from the behaviourist tradition during the 1960s. He was initially interested in social influences on behaviour and conducted a series of classic experiments during the 1960s on aggressive behaviour in children. In these experiments children imitated, without prompting or incentive, aggressive adult behaviour towards a large blow-up doll (Bandura *et al.* 1961). This raised fears that have never been resolved that children might mimic aggressive or violent behaviour seen on television.

Bandura's experiments went further in demonstrating that children do not just learn from the consequences of their own actions, but are capable of copying or modelling their behaviour on that of others. Further, he showed that they are capable of judging the likely consequences of their own actions by observing the consequences for others. Bandura's work on modelling or imitative learning has filled important gaps in explaining the speed of human learning. It also highlighted the importance and influence of the social environment on behaviour.

When Anna went on her first surgical ward placement, she had little idea of what to expect. She had previously spent time as a health care assistant in a medical ward and had received training in basic nursing skills, but still felt very nervous. Almost without thinking, she observed what other members of staff were doing; the way they made beds, took observations, communicated with patients, responded to other members of staff, the way they wore their uniform and even the way they walked. Some of the things staff did were not as she had been taught. In particular, they did not wash their hands as meticulously as she had been shown, but she nevertheless modelled her own behaviour on theirs.

The concept of modelling goes some way to explaining the process that sociologists refer to as 'socialization'. It can be seen in the way that children and adults learn new social skills and competencies. This is why practical learning is so important and why social or organizational behaviour patterns are particularly resistant to change.

Self-efficacy

Bandura (1977a, 1977b) was critical of Skinner's assertions that human behaviour is passively driven by external forces, although he acknowledged that these are influential. He argued that we all learn to monitor our own performance and reward ourselves by internal praise for good performance. The failure to recognize and reward ourselves for good performance can lead to depression. Bandura suggested that talented people often become depressed because they set themselves standards of achievement that are too high.

Bandura proposed that once children have learned to imitate a new skill, they are capable of monitoring and adjusting their own performance through a process of self-regulation, by comparing their own performance with that of others. Through this active process, they achieve a sense of self-efficacy. This refers to the fact that they have mastered the task and feel confident they can do it again. It therefore fits well with the notion of control. Indeed, Bandura (1997) referred to self-efficacy as the exercise of control.

Bandura defined perceived self-efficacy as 'beliefs in one's capabilities to organize and execute the courses of action required to produce given attainments' (Bandura 1997: 3). In other words, it refers to having self-confidence in one's ability to achieve what is wanted or needed.

He argued that our sense of self-esteem is based on the belief in our ability to achieve control, either individually or collectively. Bandura has written extensively on the concept of self-efficacy in relation to health and other life situations (Bandura 1997). Self-efficacy has been shown to be an important predictor of successful outcome in self-management programmes for chronic disease. For example, findings from a study by Lefebvre *et al.* (1999) of rheumatoid arthritis patients suggest that self-efficacy is a useful indicator of daily pain, mood and the perceived effectiveness of strategies for coping with pain.

Locus of control

Locus of control refers to a relatively stable set of beliefs about responsibility for control over outcomes. It combines the behavioural emphasis on the importance of outcomes with the principles of attribution theory (Chapter 2). Rotter (1966) developed a measure of locus of control that remains popular with researchers.

Rotter's locus of control scale placed beliefs about control on a single **bipolar** dimension: internal versus external. Internal locus of control refers to the belief that I am responsible for the things that happen to me. External locus of control refers to the belief that things that happen to me are a consequence of luck, fate, chance or someone else. This was quickly applied in health care situations. It was used, for example, to judge the likelihood that an individual would want to take responsibility for their own health and manage their own illness.

Levenson (1974) identified that there are, in fact, three independent dimensions to locus of control: internal, external (powerful others) and external (chance). Accordingly, Ken and Barbara Wallston and colleagues developed a multidimensional health locus of control measure (Wallston *et al.* 1978).

- Internal locus of control reflects the belief that my health is a consequence of my own actions.
- External (powerful others) locus of control reflects the belief that health and illness are the responsibility of others such as doctors.
- External (chance) locus of control reflects the belief that being well and getting ill is a matter luck, fate or chance.

This led to many studies to test the prediction that internal locus of control is associated with better health outcomes. To some extent the prediction was upheld. For example, a longitudinal six-year study (Wallhagen *et al.* 1994) found that internal locus of control was related to placing importance on good health. However, other findings have proved weak and inconclusive.

It soon became evident that control beliefs are not necessarily **generalized** to all situations, but need to be judged in relation to specific situations or medical conditions. For example, I may believe that my headache is under my control, but my abdominal pain is a matter for the doctor. Therefore, a variety of condition-specific locus of control measures have been devised for the purposes of research. Examples include addiction, diabetes, cancer, pain and heart disease locus of control (Walker 2001).

It has also become apparent that locus of control should not be regarded as a personality variable, but as a set of expectations that can and do change with experience. Locus of control is a useful concept in clinical practice since it gives some indication of the likelihood of people's wishes and intentions to take responsibility for their health or manage their illness. It can often be detected by observing what people do and the way they speak.

Janice has a strong internal locus of control. She likes to be well informed and searches the internet for information before seeking medical treatment. She likes to know what she can do to help herself and feels quite angry if her needs for information and explanations are not being taken seriously by the doctor. She likes to take responsibility for self-managing her symptoms when she is ill, but does not always follow the doctor's advice if she does not agree with it.

Margaret has a strong external (powerful other) locus of control and seeks medical advice whenever she has a slight illness. She always follows the doctor's advice, but finds it difficult to adhere to medication in the longer term, since this requires internal or personal control.

Mark has chance locus of control and tends to be fatalistic about his illnesses. He believes that what will be will be. Therefore he lacks the motivation to follow health advice. He is not good at monitoring his diabetes or other symptoms and, as a result, is at risk of a poorer health outcome.

Wallston (1992) subsequently argued that external chance locus of control does indeed represent the opposing pole to internal locus of control (as Rotter originally proposed), and that internal versus external (chance) locus of control is the most relevant predictor of health outcomes. There is now a good deal of evidence from research in primary and secondary health prevention to suggest that a belief in luck, fate or chance is an important predictor of poor health outcomes (Norman and Bennett 1995). We return to the concept of control in Chapter 7 on stress and coping, and Chapter 8 on health behaviours.

Cognitive behavioural therapy

Cognitive behavioural therapy (CBT) has become the most popular psychological intervention for disorders that involve anxiety. CBT, as the name suggests, combines social cognitive and behavioural treatment strategies and is based on cognitive and behavioural psychology. CBT programmes vary; most are based on group therapy and include aspects of the following, depending on the nature of the condition or problem.

- Based on behavioural psychology, CBT includes behavioural and social behavioural interventions such as progressive muscle relaxation and systematic desensitization, modelling, behaviour rehearsal, assertive training, contingency management (monitoring and manipulating antecedents and consequences), stimulus control and self-control techniques.
- Based on cognitive psychology, therapy includes cognitive restructuring. This involves reinterpreting events as less threatening and making positive self-statements such as 'I can do this'. Therapy also encourages the sharing of problem-focused coping strategies and stress management (Chapter 8). It aims to reduce fatalistic beliefs and encourage people to take control over important aspects of their lives.
- Based on humanistic psychology, there is evidence that therapist warmth and positive regard, and the establishment of a therapeutic alliance, increase patient confidence and disposition to change (Keijsers *et al.* 2000).

CBT is typically a brief intervention that involves six to ten sessions of one to two hours of problem-focused intervention. There is evidence to support the effectiveness of CBT in relation to a number of conditions that involve anxiety and depression, including chronic pain.

> Morley *et al.* (1999) reported a systematic review and meta-analysis of CBT compared to control treatments and no treatment for chronic pain. Compared to waiting-list control, CBT was associated with a moderate level of improvement on all measures. Compared to alternative active treatments, CBT produced significantly greater changes in pain experience, cognitive coping and appraisal (positive coping measures), and reduced behavioural expression of pain, but not depression, cognitive appraisals or coping, and social role functioning. The authors concluded that CBT was an effective treatment for the management of chronic pain.

Other systematic reviews show behaviour therapy or CBT to be effective in the management of chronic low back pain (van Tulder *et al.* 2003), chronic fatigue syndrome (Price and Couper 2003) and schizophrenia (Paley and Shapiro 2002). However while CBT has been shown to lead to clinical improvements, there is no clear research-based evidence that it is any more effective than other psychological interventions for depression (Parker *et al.* 2003).

Applying behavioural principles to designing a health education programme

Cognitive behavioural therapy can also be used to change health-related behaviours. An example of such a programme is the 'Quit for life' smoking cessation programme designed and tested by David Marks (see Marks *et al.* 2000). The programme incorporates issues raised earlier in this chapter, including principles of counter-conditioning (substituting reinforcing alternatives), stimulus control and reinforcement management. The key assumptions on which this is based are as follows.

- Nicotine has immediate positive reinforcing consequences for the smoker: it is relaxing, increases alertness and improves cognitive performance (because of these effects, smoking provides a useful way of coping with stress).
- Smoking a cigarette fills time. This provides thinking time for problem solving, and 'time out' from difficult situations.
- Smoking suppresses appetite. Eating often replaces smoking, but leads to weight gain (many people relapse because they gain weight)
- Smoking is a social activity and the smoker is often under peer pressure to smoke. Peer approval is reinforcing; peer disapproval acts as a punisher.

- Lighting up is a habit that takes place in certain situations without thinking (e.g. having a cup of coffee or after a meal). Smoking is under stimulus control.

The following techniques were designed as part of the programme to address these points. Will power plays no part in this programme and the individual does not pledge to stop smoking. Smoking behaviour declines naturally as the programme is implemented.

1. Interrupt the habitual element of smoking by putting a rubber band round the packet that must first be removed. Reduce the association of cigarettes with pleasure: place a personal message under the rubber band and read it out each time a cigarette is drawn out. For example:

> This cigarette is making me ill
> I do not like this cigarette
> I do not wish to smoke this cigarette

The individual *must* then take out a cigarette and smoke it so that a subconscious association is gradually built up between the cigarette and something unpleasant.

2. Reduce the habitual effect by identifying the situations in which the patient tends to light up without thinking and placing another message under the rubber band to read out before lighting the cigarette in that situation:

> Just because I have had a meal, I do not need to smoke
> Next time I finish a meal, I will not want to smoke

3. Find new ways of keeping the hands occupied, such as doodling or worry beads.
4. Build in an exercise and weight-control programme to prevent excessive weight gain.
5. Rehearse assertive skills for saying 'no' to peers.
6. Find social support from others who do not smoke. Marks included a 'buddy' system. Each participant was paired with another person in the programme whom they could phone if they were finding things too hard or felt they might give in to temptation.
7. Find alternative methods of stress management, for example relaxation, yoga.

The success rate at the end of a year for the self-help version of this programme, reported by Marks *et al.* (2000), was 25%, making it 26 times more cost-effective than nicotine replacement therapy.

Summary of key points

- Behaviour and behaviour change is influenced by its antecedents, and its consequences provided these are desirable, immediate and certain.

- Classical conditioning theory may help to prevent, explain and treat many common fears, phobias and other symptoms such as nausea or allergic responses that are associated with intense physiological arousal.
- Many health-related and illness behaviours appear to be habits that are under stimulus control, rather than cognitive control.
- The theory of learned helplessness suggests that depression is caused by the experience of perceived loss of control.
- Self-efficacy is an important predictor of positive health outcomes; chance locus of control is an important predictor of adverse health outcomes.
- Cognitive behavioural therapy is a popular and effective intervention for the management of many chronic disorders and can also be used to help people change health-related behaviours such as smoking.

Further reading

Conner, M. and Norman, P. (eds.) (1995) *Predicting health behaviour.* Buckingham: Open University Press, Chapters 3 and 6.

Marks, D.F., Murray, M., Evans, B. and Willig, C. (2000) *Health Psychology: Theory, Research and Practice.* London, Sage, Chapter 8.

Mirowsky, J. and Ross, C.E. (2003) *Social Causes of Psychological Distress,* 2nd edition. New York: Aldine de Gruyter.

CHAPTER FIVE

DEVELOPMENT AND CHANGE ACROSS THE LIFESPAN

- What are children of different ages able to understand about health and illness?
- How can we explain complex issues to children of different ages?
- Why are attachment relationships so important, and what is the impact of separation?
- How might parenting influence health-related behaviours?
- What is important when considering development across the lifespan?
- What is special about the psychology of later life?
- How do people respond to loss?
- How can we help people to resolve grief and retain hope in the face of loss?

Introduction

This chapter examines aspects of development and change from early in life until the end of life. It starts by examining cognitive and social development, drawing upon some classic psychological theory and research. Cognitive development refers to development of thinking and understanding about the world. The concept of social development centres on social relationships and includes the growth of close relationships with others. The chapter moves on to consider theories of development across the lifespan, focusing particularly on later life. We complete the chapter by considering issues related to loss.

The development of thinking and understanding

People develop both cognitively and socially throughout their lives, though psychological research has tended to focus particularly upon early infancy and childhood. Our understanding of cognitive development during this period has been informed by two key theorists and theories, which we consider in some depth: Piaget's theory of cognitive development and Vygotsky's sociocultural theory of cognitive development.

Piaget's theory of cognitive development

Until the 1930s, children were believed to be small versions of adults. It was believed that they thought the same way as adults but had less knowledge because of their lack of experience. Piaget (1929) helped to change this notion. He also challenged existing behaviourist approaches to development which proposed that children learn largely though reward and punishment (Chapter 4). Jean Piaget was a Swiss psychologist who studied in the psychoanalytic school and became very interested in the way children's thinking developed. Based on observations and experiments, mainly with his own children, he produced a theory of cognitive development that has had a profound influence on education and research into people's understandings.

At the centre of Piaget's theory is the concept of cognitive structures, which he called schemas (see also Chapters 2 and 4). A schema in this context can be viewed as an organized collection of memories, actions and strategies that enable us to predict and understand the world around us (Keenan 2002). According to Piaget, four key processes are involved in establishing schemas: 'adapting', 'organizing', 'assimilation' and 'accommodation'. The individual is viewed as adapting to new information and events in the environment and organizing this information into a coherent form. 'Assimilation' refers to the process of taking information into existing schemas, stored in the brain. The existing schema is then altered or modified to accommodate this new information.

Piaget (1963) argued that children progress through a series of four main stages in order to reach the stage of adult understanding. The main features of these four stages of development are summarized below.

0–2 years: the 'sensori-motor' stage
- Infants use sensory information gained through the mouth and hands to learn about the properties of objects.
- From about 6 months, children learn that objects remain the same when they are out of sight. Games of hide and seek encourage this discovery.
- From about 18 months, children are able to use symbolic thought. This means that one object can be used to represent another in play and language is used to represent thought.

2–7 years: the 'pre-operational' stage
- Children remain 'egocentric'. This means that they are unable to see things from the perspectives of others.
- Children attach human attributes to inanimate objects.
- Children are unable to 'conserve' the properties of objects. This means, for example, they tend identify a short fat glass as containing less water than a long thin one, even when they have seen the same amount of water poured from one to the other.

7–12 years: the 'concrete operational' stage
• Children learn about the conservation of properties such as volume and
  are able to deal with most abstract concepts.

12+ years: the 'formal operational' stage
• Children are now capable of adult reasoning.

The key features of Piaget's theory are that these stages are both invariant
and universal. 'Invariant' means that the child progresses through them in
a set order, and no stage can be missed out. 'Universal' means that the same
sequence of learning occurs in all children, irrespective of their social or
cultural background. The stage theory does, however, allow that the speed
of progress through the stages might be influenced by inherited traits,
increase in the capacity of working memory, or environmental factors
(Keenan 2002).

Piaget's theory has been extremely influential and stimulated a large
amount of research, though more recent researchers have challenged
his ideas. The main areas of criticism focus upon the nature of the experiments used. His critics argue that Piaget's experiments were too complex or unfamiliar for children, and their responses may have led him to
underestimate their abilities within his stages of development.

The best-known example of Piaget's experiments is the 'three mountains'
experiment (Piaget and Inhelder 1956), which appeared to demonstrate
that young children are unable to see things (literally) from the
perspectives of others. Piaget termed this 'egocentrism'. The child was
seated in front of a table, on which was a model of three mountains, and
told that there was a doll on the other side of the table. They were then
shown a selection of photographs and asked to choose the photograph of
the view the doll was likely to see.

The 'three mountains' experiment may be criticized for its poor ecological validity. Outside of mountainous countries like Switzerland where
Piaget worked, mountains are not part of children's normal experience.
Margaret Donaldson later illustrated how children are able to see things
from someone else's perspective at a much younger age than Piaget predicted, provided the experiment uses more familiar objects. For example,
Martin Hughes asked children to hide a 'naughty teddy' behind some building bricks so that the 'policeman' doll could not see it (Donaldson 1978).
Experiments with children always need to be interpreted with caution
because it is often quite difficult to tell if they report what they really
believe, or what they think adults want to hear. Further experiments using
dolls led Donaldson to confirm that children of this age can find it difficult
to know what other people see from their different positions. However,

they are much better at understanding how other people feel and what they might be thinking or planning to do (Donaldson 1990). Therefore, children at a pre-operational stage cannot be truly held to be 'egocentric'.

Piaget's work generated a large volume of research into children's understanding, some of which concerned aspects of health, illnesses, knowledge of their bodies and death. However, more recently, many psychological theorists have become disenchanted with the rigidity of stage theories and have sought alternative explanations for development and adaptation in a complex world.

Vygotsky's sociocultural theory of cognitive development

More recent developmental theorists, led by Vygotsky, have tended to focus not on cognitive stages but on the influences of the social context in which learning takes place. Vygotsky was a Russian contemporary of Piaget, but his work was little known in the West until more recently. Like Piaget, Vygotsky (1978) viewed children as actively exploring and interacting with the world around them. But while Piaget largely seemed to view this as a solitary activity, Vygotsky was interested in the role of social interaction and language in the child's development. Vygotsky argued that children are particularly likely to learn from others when there is a small gap between what the child can achieve on their own and what they could do with the collaboration or guidance of someone else who is more skilled. Vygotsky used the term 'zone of proximal development' to describe this gap. Essentially, it means that the child learns 'one small step at a time, with help and guidance'.

Lee was having difficulty opening a box and was getting very frustrated. Jo observed that the cause of Lee's frustration was his failure to understand which was the top and which was the bottom. If Jo had assumed that Lee was not old enough to open the box for himself, he might have taken it and opened it for him. Instead, Jo showed Lee where he was going wrong, and then gently guided him while he did it himself. In this way, Lee learned an additional skill that would enable him to open the box for himself in future.

The concept of the 'zone of proximal development' has been very influential in education. For example, it has led to the introduction of peer teaching, where those who are more skilled are encouraged to teach those at a slightly lower level of skill development. Jerome Bruner (1983) subsequently used the term 'scaffolding' to describe the interactive process whereby the adult modifies the amount of help and guidance they give in relation to the child's responses so that the child can achieve more and more. An important feature of Vygotsky's theory is that, unlike Piaget's theory, it has no upper age or stage limit, and this principle can also be applied to adult learning (Chapter 8).

Vygotsky's theory enables us to explain the effect of cultural influences and differences on the development of understanding. Unlike Piaget's stage theory which proposed that progression takes place in a rigid sequence, Vygotsky's theory indicates that the child is able to develop in a more flexible way. Thus, they may attain a greater understanding in some areas than others, because of their different social opportunities to engage with and receive guidance from others. This helps us to understand why children with health problems often appear to be so far advanced developmentally in their knowledge about their body, illness, drugs or procedures.

Children's knowledge of their bodies

It is clearly useful to take account of children's understanding when preparing them for medical procedures, offering health advice or gaining consent. Piaget's theory predicts that children's understanding relates to their developmental level, which roughly equates to their age. In contrast, Vygotsky predicts that understanding will vary according to experience and opportunities to interact with knowledgeable others. The following study (an important one at the time) illustrates how children's understandings of their bodies and concepts of illness are likely to be different from those of adults.

Eiser and Patterson (1983) interviewed groups of healthy children aged 6, 8, 10 and 12 years about what was inside their bodies and what these parts were for. All of the children knew that the mouth and stomach were involved in eating but few were aware of digestive processes or that food was absorbed into the bloodstream. Some 6-year-olds did not know what organs were involved in breathing although, with increasing age, the heart and lungs were mentioned more frequently. Most of the children knew that arms and legs were needed for swimming, however, younger children related this to the bones while 54% of 12-year-olds talked about the role of the brain in controlling activity.

It certainly appears that younger children have a much more rudimentary understanding of the location and function of body parts. However, there is wide variation in the level of knowledge regardless of age. Some young children are quite sophisticated in their understanding, while those working in health care will be aware how rudimentary the knowledge of many adults is about the inner workings of their bodies. These types of observation later led Eiser to refute the Piagetian interpretation of their findings. The important thing, according to Vytogsky, is to find out what the child already knows and to build on that.

Children's understanding of health and illness

If the child's ability to think and understand is limited by their stage of cognitive development, it is expected that their understanding of health and illness will correspond to their developmental stage.

In a study regarded by many as seminal, Bibace and Walsh (1981) asked children to describe how people catch a cold. They used Piaget's developmental framework to interpret their findings and identified a six-stage model of children's understanding of illness that corresponded to their age. At an early age, children tended to believe that colds are caused by external forces such as the sun and, slightly later, magic. Later, they acquired the notion that colds are caught from contact with other people or from breathing cold air. From the age of about 11, the children were more likely to explain illness in terms of malfunctioning organs and causes such as germs or viruses. From the age of about 16, adolescents started to appreciate that people exposed to viruses might catch cold if they were more susceptible, for example if they were run down.

The findings of this study appear to support the view that children gradually become more sophisticated in their understanding. Bibace and Walsh took their findings as evidence that children cannot understand an explanation of illness in advance of their stage of cognitive development. However, Vygotsky's theory predicts that their understanding will relate more to the types of explanations that children are provided with.

Veldtman *et al.* (2000) sought to evaluate knowledge and understanding of their illnesses in children and adolescents, aged between 7 and 18 years, who had congenital and acquired heart disease. They found that less than one-third had a good understanding of their illness; 77% did not know the medical name of their condition, and 33% had a wrong or poor understanding of their illness. Even some older adolescents had an entirely wrong concept of their disease. Of particular importance is their finding that understanding was not directly related to age.

Rushforth (1999) reviewed the available evidence in order to enhance information-giving and consent-taking. She proposed that children's understanding is often related to the explanations they have been given. For example, in relation to pain, they are more likely to be able to explain why an injection hurts than why they have a headache. She suggested that this is because adults are more likely to spend time explaining an injection. She also pointed out ambiguities in the English language that can lead children to make misinterpretations. She gave the example of ivy (instead of IV).

She argued that many childhood fears related to illness may have their origins in such simple misconceptions. Therefore, it is essential to check the child's understanding before giving further information.

This type of research tells us that it is essential to give explanations at a level that each individual child is able to understand. Before the age of about 7, it may be helpful to use dolls to enable them to illustrate what they think is going on. It is essential to check with parents what words children use to describe certain body parts or functions and to check out what the child has understood. It is also important to remember to check out exactly what the child has understood about what he or she has been told, and to support the parents to deal with children's questions.

Sasha has been trying to explain to Lee that she is expecting another baby. She has told him that there is a baby growing in mummy's tummy. But when Lee asked how the baby got in there, Sasha was not sure what to say. It is unlikely, at the age of 4, that he will be able to understand an abstract concept such as conception. There are some very good books that help to explain pregnancy and childbirth to young children, and Sasha has decided to get one from the library next time she is in town. This will enable her to find out what Lee already knows and help her to provide the 'scaffolding' around which he can develop his learning on this subject.

Children's understanding of death and dying

According to Piaget's theory, children at the pre-operational stage of development may find it impossible to accept the permanence of death.

Lee has a friend, James, also aged 4, whose father was recently killed in a road accident. His mother told him that his daddy had died, and James was later taken to visit the grave. But a few weeks after that, he said to his mother 'Please can we go and dig daddy up?'.

Meadows (1993) suggested that most children are unable to accept the permanence of death until they are about 9 years old. Rushforth (1999) suggested that they are may be unable to accept death in terms of the impact on the family until adolescence. However, Rushforth argued that the greatest disservice we do children is to try to protect them from the realities of events such as death. In seeking to fill gaps in their knowledge, their imagination may be far worse than reality. It is worth reflecting that even adults have difficulty in accepting death as permanent unless or until they have seen the body or obtained concrete evidence of the death. An abstract concept such as death may be more easily understood and ultimately less frightening if learned about through the death of a pet, provided family members are themselves willing to confront the reality of death. We deal further with the concept of loss later in this chapter.

The importance of play

Play is an important part in the life of the developing child as it provides opportunities for learning and enables the child to gain mastery over important skills, including social skills. Play begins when babies repeat acts that they find pleasurable, or which have a direct effect on their environment and those in it. Piaget (1951) argued that play enables babies to practice motor, cognitive and social competencies. Both Piaget and Vygotsky noted that children use symbolic or pretend play to act out different roles and situations. This enables them to learn to cope with a variety of possible situations, including emotional crises, interpersonal conflicts and social roles. For example, playing at doctors and nurses, or mothers and fathers, is a good way to learn about different aspects of the social world in which they live. Play is a useful way of preparing children for medical procedures and can also be useful in preparing children for life-changing events.

Sasha has been encouraging Lee to play at mothers and fathers with his friend, in preparation for the birth of his new brother or sister. Boys are often discouraged from paying with dolls, but Sasha has provided him with an old doll of hers that cries and wets its nappy. She hopes that he will be better prepared and less jealous once the baby is born. Meanwhile, Jo has been encouraging Lee to play football and other 'boys' games' to build up a special type of relationship between stepfather and son and distract from the extra attention required by the new baby.

Children's social development

This section is concerned with the development of important social relationships during the life of the child, starting at birth. Relationships that involve a close emotional bond with other people or things (such as pets or acquisitions), whenever these occur in life, are termed **attachment** relationships.

Attachment

The human infant is dependent on adults for all its needs in the early years. Therefore, there are good reasons why babies need to establish a close relationship with their mother or caregiver. The early behaviourist operant conditioning view was that attachment to the mother occurred because she provided reinforcement in the form of food and comfort. This explanation was discounted when Harlow's famous experiments with rhesus monkeys (Harlow 1959) demonstrated that a baby monkey preferred soft physical contact with an inanimate object, even when it did not deliver milk. Harlow's studies also confirmed that female monkeys who had no experience of mothering subsequently neglected or abused their own children. These experiments identified attachment as an important requisite for normal social development.

Based on observations of other species, psychologists believed that there might be a critical sensitive period soon after birth when it was essential for mother and baby to 'bond'. Klaus and Kennell (1976) studied the effect of increased infant–mother contact soon after birth and found that close contact at birth stimulated caring responses in the mother. As a result, maternity units were encouraged to facilitate this process. Certainly, babies are able to recognize their mother's smell and learn to distinguish her face soon after they are born. However, Rutter (1979) noted the propensity of adoptive parents to develop strong attachments with older babies and cast doubt on the notion of a sensitive period for attachment. Babies do need to develop strong attachment relationship with their principle caregivers, but this may take place at any time during the early weeks or months.

Attachment in infants refers to 'a relationship between caregiver and infant that takes most of the infant's first year to develop. . . . [It is] considered to be long lasting (perhaps for years), but it is changing in nature' (Damon 1983: 29). The name most closely associated with investigations of attachment in human infants is John Bowlby. Bowlby (1969) noted that human babies exhibit a number of behaviours that have survival value because they engage the adults who will meet their needs. These include signalling behaviour (crying, cooing, babbling and smiling) and approach behaviour (clinging, non-nutritional sucking, and maintaining eye contact with the caregiver). Bowlby's theory of attachment is based on an interactional model. This means that attachment is not dependent solely on the infant's or mother's responses. Rather, each influences the other. Therefore, a depressed mother who is unable adequately to respond to the infant's demands for attention may influence the baby's subsequent behaviour by failing to respond to signals like crying. Likewise, a very small pre-term infant may be unable to produce responses like crying or smiling that elicit adult attention. Bowlby has suggested that primary attachment is important in infancy because it provides the template for subsequent intimate and social relationships.

Separation

By the age of between 7 and 12 months, Bowlby noted that babies become very distressed in the absence of their mother or primary caregiver. They become very wary of strangers and protest vigorously. He termed this 'separation anxiety'. Bowlby emphasized that separation from the primary caregiver before the age of 5 years might damage the mental health of the child. His research was used to argue that women should not go out to work and leave their babies with other caregivers. However, more recent studies have identified that attachment to multiple caregivers is possible. There is no evidence of adverse effects of other childcare arrangements on the child, provided stable and good-quality alternative sources of care are provided (Schaffer 1988).

Until the 1960s, it was common when a child was admitted to hospital for the mother to be asked to leave the child and stay away. This was because children were observed to become extremely distressed each time their mothers had to leave. James Robertson worked closely with Bowlby in the late 1940s, and later made a series of harrowing films that revealed the extent and characteristics of distress shown by separated young children (Robertson and Robertson 1967–73). The stages of separation were marked by protest (anger and loud crying), despair (withdrawal and less vigorous crying) and, later, detachment (the child outwardly displayed cheerful behaviour but remained emotionally distant). As a result, children's units reversed their policies and now encourage mothers to stay, if possible, for the duration of the child's admission.

Types of attachment

It was observed that not all children respond in the same way when separated from their mothers. This led to a series of experiments into different types of attachment relationships and their effects on separation.

During the 1970s, Mary Ainsworth conducted a series of classic experiments on the nature of attachment and stranger fear, called the 'strange situation experiment' (Ainsworth *et al.* 1978). This involved a series of prescribed events that took place in one room. The activity and reaction of the infant was recorded.

The mother and her infant enter the observation room that contains toys. The mother puts the child to play with the toys and sits down. In this situation, the child initially stays close to the mother, then explores the toys, occasionally returning to the mother to regain contact. This implies that the child sees the mother as a safe base from which to explore.

Then a strange person comes into the room and talks to the mother. The child returns to the mother and clings to her or hides behind her to peep out at the stranger. After a short time, most children in this situation return to play with the toys, though some continue to cling to the mother.

Then the mother leaves the room, leaving the child with the stranger. Ainsworth noted that most children immediately stopped playing. Most cried and the remainder showed signs of disturbance. Some went to the door to try to get out and waited there for the mother's return. Others remained in one spot on the floor holding onto a toy.

Ainsworth found that the age of maximum separation anxiety to be about 1 year. She observed variations in the type of response, depending on the nature of the attachment relationship with the mother. She recorded three main types of attachment (Ainsworth *et al.* 1978):

Secure attachment (approx. 66%). The child plays happily with the toys, reacts positively to strangers and returns to play. Play is reduced during the mother's absence and the child is distressed. On the mother's return, the child seeks contact and then returns to play.

Avoidant attachment or unattached (approx. 20%). The child plays with toys, unaffected by the mother's whereabouts in the room. The child is not distressed on separation and, on the mother's return, the child ignores her or may move away. If the child is distressed, they are as easily comforted by the stranger as by the mother.

Resistant attachment (approx. 10–12%). The child is fussy and wary in the mother's presence and has difficulty leaving her. On her return, the child seeks contact, but at the same time struggles against the mother and appears angry. The child remains uninvolved in play.

Subsequent research sought to identify features of parenting associated with these styles of response. The mothers of children who were securely attached appeared more responsive, showed more affection, including touching, smiling and praise, and more social stimulation. Those whose children showed avoidant attachment or insecure attachment showed much lower levels of these types of interaction. Follow-up studies have indicated that securely attached children are more likely to be initiators of play as well as active participants in play, more curious and eager to learn, and showed more empathy towards other children. Those who have insecure attachment relationships tend to be socially withdrawn and less curious (Maccoby 1980). But Maccoby noted that (at least until the age of 3), insecure relationships can change if the quality of the parental response improves. This offers important support for the idea of parenting classes.

Teenage motherhood is associated with economic and social problems, including a higher incidence of low-birthweight babies. Concerns are frequently expressed about the quality of parenting. American nursing researchers, Spieker and Bensley (1994) studied 197 adolescent mother–infant pairs to identify factors that influenced their parenting. They examined the relationship with teenage mothers' own mothers, living arrangements, and the type of attachment shown by the infants. Their results showed that infants were more likely to be securely attached if their mothers lived with their partners and had a high level of social support from their own mothers. If the teenage parent's mother did not provide support, the infant seemed to do better when their mother lived independently, rather than with her partner. Cause and effect is difficult to establish in a correlational study, but these findings may indicate that, while a teenage mother benefits from advice and support, it is difficult for her to display parenting behaviours towards her child in the presence of her own mother.

It is important to note that the quality of the attachment relationship reflects a two-way interaction. The temperamental disposition of the child may affect the mother's behaviour, just as the mother's behaviour may affect the responses of the child. For example, some babies resist being held and cuddled and it may be difficult for the mother to form a secure attachment relationship with such a child.

Moral reasoning and development

The development of moral reasoning in children is important because it is associated with independence of thought and action, and the ability to resist peer pressure.

Kohlberg was interested in how children learn to tell right from wrong. He studied how boys from the age of 10 dealt with moral dilemmas such as theft and criminal damage (Kohlberg 1969). He found that younger children conformed to adult rules, but they determined the goodness or badness of an act by its consequences. They tended to reason that if it is possible to 'get away with it', then it could not be very bad. Older children tended to obey the rules of their social group in order to gain praise and avoid censure, but, by the age of 16, adolescents tended to demonstrate commitment to a set of principles shared with a reference group. In contrast, the highest level of adult moral reasoning involves the development of a self-chosen moral code and set of ethical principles.

Based on these observations, Kohlberg developed a stage theory of moral reasoning. Although stage theories are no longer accepted, these observations have clear implications for the ways in which issues such as smoking, drug-taking and alcohol consumption need to be dealt with in relation to adolescent boys (though it might be different for girls). Young boys need careful monitoring to make sure that they do not 'get away with it', but are likely to respond to adult codes. Peer pressure is a strong influence on teenage behaviours and is likely to take priority over 'rational' medical arguments. Health messages that appeal to adult reason may have little or no effect if the teenager belongs to a social group that rejects them.

Parenting styles

In considering the development of moral reasoning, it is of interest to examine the effect of child-rearing on children's behaviour. Baumrind (1971) conducted a series of studies in which she tested the relationship between parents' behaviour and various characteristics of the children. She identified three distinct types of parenting:

> Authoritative parents are characterized as setting reasonable standards and enforcing them firmly and consistently but without physical punishment. They expect the child to conform to those standards, but provide explanations, guidance and feedback, and encourage self-direction.
> Authoritarian parents expect obedience. They set absolute standards, often using physical punishment. They attempt to control the attitudes as well as the behaviour of the child and discourage argument.
> Permissive parents behave in a positive and accepting way towards the child's impulses, desires and actions and make little attempt to regulate the child's behaviour. They attempt reasoning, but avoid any exercise of control and make few demands on the child.

Baumrind (1967) explored the effects of parenting styles on the child. Findings suggest that the children of authoritative parents tend to be more independent, more self-directed and more socially responsible. The children of authoritarian parents tend to show less independence, develop external **locus of control**, lack empathy and have lower self-esteem (Coopersmith 1967). The children of permissive parents tend to be more immature, lack social responsibility and are not particularly independent. A more recent longitudinal study by Baumrind (1991) suggested that parents who used an authoritative style may be more successful in protecting their children from problem drug use, as opposed to casual recreational use, in adolescence.

> Cohen *et al.* (1994) conducted a large four-year prospective survey of pre-adolescents to identify which specific parenting behaviours were associated with the onset of alcohol and tobacco use. They found that children who claimed their parents spent more time with them and communicated with them more frequently had lower rates of alcohol and tobacco use. The findings indicate strong influences of parental monitoring and positive relationships on adolescent vulnerability to peer pressure and subsequent substance use. As a result, the authors

recommend that parenting education with respect to substance use should take place before their children reach adolescence.

Important dimensions of parenting for boys and girls appear to be emotional warmth and parental involvement, particularly in protecting against depression (Taris and Bok 1996). There are indications in the literature of gender differences in aspects of parenting associated with health risk. For example, Taris and Bok found that, in young adults, the father's involvement was linked to having an internal locus of control (Chapter 4). However, the opposite effect was found for over-involvement of the mother. Young adults who felt unable to influence what happened to them were more likely to feel depressed. Griffin *et al.* (2000) confirmed that parental monitoring is associated with lower levels of alcohol use in boys but not girls. It appears important not to assume that the behaviour patterns of males and females are the same or have the same effect.

Development across the lifespan

People continue to develop throughout their whole lifespan, and not just during childhood as the developmental theories of Freud and Piaget might lead one to believe. People continue to learn and adapt to new experiences throughout their lives. Social lives and social identities develop and change throughout the lifespan. The next section briefly introduces two prominent theories of lifespan development: Erikson's psychosocial development and Levinson's life stage model.

Drawing on psychoanalytic theory, Erikson (1980) developed an eight-stage model of psychosocial development. He proposed that at each stage of development, special psychological tasks need to be achieved in order to overcome developmental challenges or crises and allow development to proceed successfully. Successful accomplishment of these tasks results in **adaptation** and failure in maladaptation. For example, in the first year of life the baby needs to develop a trusting relationship with another person, usually the mother; and if the relationship is established, that is considered to be a successful outcome. This is rather similar to the attachment process proposed by Bowlby. Like Piaget, Erikson (1980) proposed a series of developmental stages during childhood. Unlike Piaget, he proposed three subsequent stages:

Young adulthood (the 20s) is portrayed as a period of competition versus collaboration, during which people find new friendships and sexual partnerships.

Adulthood (30 to 50s) focuses on family life and the tasks of caring and sharing

'Old age' (50s+) is associated with a state of wisdom or despair.

Although Erikson deserves credit for being the first to consider the possibility of development and change across the lifespan, his emphasis on psychological as opposed to situational challenges is problematic and there is no evidence to support the notion of stage development. His approach failed to take account of gender differences in the challenges faced and tasks to be achieved, and his theory does not easily accommodate cultural difference or demographic change. For example, at a time when most people expect to live well into their 80s, many regard 50 as the start of middle age, bringing with it new opportunities and possibly new relationships.

Levinson *et al.* (1978) subsequently proposed an alternative stage theory based on a series of life transitions that reflect changing family and work roles across the lifespan. Levinson is perhaps best known for introducing the concept of the mid-life transition, subsequently referred to by others as the 'mid-life crisis'. However, the transitions identified by Levinson do not appear to reflect life stages. Rather they appear to represent the changing patterns of challenge and demand likely to be faced by the majority of people at different points in their lives. For example, young adults move away from home, make and break new friendships, establish and negotiate sexual relationships, get a job, start a family. In early middle life, people may have to reappraise life goals in the light of achievements, or the failure to achieve previously determined goals. This might include having or not having children, career progression or change, adjustments in lifestyle or expectations, maintaining relationships or separations, dealing with success or failure. Later middle life often includes the demands of caring for older parents, loss of parents, children leaving home (or staying at home), separation or divorce, the menopause and increasing concerns about health. These changes are probably best analysed in relation to psychological theories of the self and the self concept (Chapter 2), stress and coping (Chapter 7) and loss (later in this chapter). The exception is the body of psychology related to old age or later life.

Later life

Old age has been categorized as a separate life stage since antiquity. For example, Falkner and de Luce (1992) noted that the Greeks and Romans characterized old age as a time of physical and mental deterioration, social marginalization and closeness of death. From this, it would appear that the ageist stereotype has a long history. Nowadays, the majority of those requiring medical care and hospitalization are over the age of retirement. Therefore the needs of this group deserve particular consideration. But how should we define 'old age'?

Theories of ageing

Old age is often defined in chronological terms, and the age of retirement at 60 or 65 has commonly been used as a convenient point of entry. But these days, people retire at any point from the age of 50, and the official age of retirement is likely to rise to 70. Therefore the transition point is variable. People now live so long that is common to refer to the old as aged 80 and over. But while some people are decrepit at the age of 60, others are still working full-time well into their 90s. Therefore chronological age is not a particularly useful concept. Functional age is easier to define; yet this needs to take account of emotional, cognitive and physical functioning. Variations in the ageing process mean that old age is very difficult to define.

Traditionally, theories of old age have focused on decline. Certainly it is for many people a period of decline in physical function. Yet for most people, decline is not gradual. It is precipitated by one or a series of adverse events such illness or a fall. Decline in cognitive function is far from inevitable, especially for those who keep themselves mentally active. Cumming and Henry's (1961) disengagement theory used to be a prominent theory of old age. Based on an American study of people aged 50–90 reported in 1961, the researchers noted that retirement and other events such as death of a spouse led to a restriction in lifestyle. They characterized the older elderly as solitary, retreating into a world of memories. In the twenty-first century, people are fitter, better off financially, able to undergo joint replacements to avoid pain and incapacity, and generally enjoy a much more active retirement. These observations led to an alternative theory of ageing, activity theory (Havighurst *et al.* 1968).

But the fact is that ageing is not the same for everyone and to apply either of these theories to the whole population over 65 would be ridiculous. It is probably better to undertake an individual assessment of the person and their lifestyle. Nevertheless, there is evidence that memories of the past play an increasingly important part in adjustment as people approach the end of their lives, regardless of their age.

The life review

Reminiscence has been the focus of intensive study for those interested in the psychology of later life. Erikson (1980) characterized old age as a period of either fulfilment or despair. This may be because as people approach the end of their lives, most seem naturally to reflect on their accomplishments and try to find a sense of meaning or purpose for past problems or failures. Butler (1974) termed this natural process the 'life review' and argued that it is associated with healthy ageing. Life review therapy is a process through which the individual is encouraged to review, reorganize and re-evaluate the overall picture of their life, and gain a sense of meaning and coherence. This has been confirmed as an effective therapy for depressed older people (Bohlmeijer 2003). It can be emotionally painful remembering situations associated with shame or guilt, but Coleman (1999) has suggested that life review therapy has a 'confessional' dimension that encourages reconciliation.

Haight and Olson (1989) developed a structured format for life review therapy for use by nurses and home aides. The intervention consists of six one-hour sessions during which the older person reviews happy and sad events in childhood and middle life, and finishes with a reappraisal of these events. Structured life review has been shown to lead to improvements in life satisfaction, well-being and self-esteem, and decreases in depression.

Life review therapy should not be regarded as the preserve of old age, but may be helpful for others who have experienced important losses or face a terminal illness. It is part of a growing tradition of narrative psychology and narrative therapy that provides a means of closure, dealing with unfinished business and achieving a sense of coherence (Chapters 2 and 7). Loss is a common feature of life and is often a central feature of the life review.

Loss

Experiencing loss is an inevitable part of life. When we make choices about careers, relationships, or places and ways to live, choosing one inevitably involves loss of the other. Transitions like marriage, promotion at work and having a baby bring both gains and losses. Some losses may be not of actual things or events, but of potential events, roles or relationships, and it is therefore possible to lose something that you have never had. This is a type of loss experienced by many infertile couples, for whom the role of parent cannot be realized. Other losses, like employment, homelessness or loss of a body part or function, are more obvious.

Kelly (1998) reviewed the multiple losses associated with chronic pain and illness. Concrete losses include loss of mobility, energy, comfort, physical activity and lifestyle. Personal and interpersonal losses include loss of privacy, body image, human relationships, independence, sense of self, family roles, work roles, sexual fulfilment, ideal life and loss of life as it used to be. It can be seen from this that loss can take many forms and chronically ill or disabled patients need opportunities to come to terms with them.

The death of someone we love is generally recognized as one of the most serious adverse life events, yet loss of a pet or other attachment object can be almost as traumatic. Attachment bonds are important throughout our lives, and the disruption or breakdown of close relationships is an important source of loss, leading to physical and psychological illness, including impaired immune functioning (Chapter 7), accidents, substance abuse, suicide, depression and other forms of psychopathology (Hazan and Zeifman 1999). Nurses encounter death more frequently than most other people, but many still have a high level of anxiety about death. Payne *et al.* (1998) found that those working in emergency care settings had higher levels of death anxiety than those working in palliative care settings, possibly because they had less opportunity to discuss their feelings. The next sections consider theories that account for people's responses to loss.

Bereavement is the process surrounding loss. Grief is the reaction associated with loss. Mourning is the behavioural and emotional expression of grief. Mourning is strongly influenced by cultural norms. For example, the rituals that occur after a death, such as laying out the body, the type of funeral, and the type of clothing worn by mourners, are all very much dependent upon cultural norms. In America, it is common practice to have open coffins. This used to be common in Britain, but is no more. The funeral is often followed by a family or community gathering where the deceased individual is remembered and aspects of his or her life celebrated. It is probably helpful to have well-accepted rituals because they direct people as to how to behave and how to respond to each other during a time when it is difficult to make informed decisions. Rituals, such as state funerals, both contain and allow public expression of feelings. Rituals also mark the status change of individuals, such as a wife becoming a widow. They provide an opportunity to demonstrate emotional support, and enable grieving people to derive comfort from others.

Traditional theories of loss and grief

Traditional theories of loss, like attachment, were derived from psychoanalysis, because the key theorists in this area emerged from that tradition. Central to these is the concept of 'ego defence', which means that some things that happen are so threatening that the conscious mind, the ego, cannot cope with them. Freud introduced the notion of defence mechanisms, which are unconscious ways of coping. Defence mechanisms, such as denial, may be helpful in allowing us to continue functioning in very stressful situations, so that we can 'work through' problems at a later stage. Freud suggested that in order to recover from loss, we need to confront our fears and feelings in a conscious process that he called 'grief work'. Freud suggested that failure to do this might lead to prolonged or pathological types of grief. This has led to an emphasis on the importance of bereavement counselling. However, Jordan and Neimeyer (2003), having studied the literature on bereavement intervention, concluded that the scientific basis for accepting the efficacy of grief counselling appears weak (see also the section on post-traumatic stress in Chapter 7).

Two of the best-known models used to understand grief and bereavement are those described by Elisabeth Kübler-Ross and Colin Murray Parkes. These models were both based on clinical observations. Kübler-Ross (1969) based her stage model of loss on her clinical experiences with dying patients who were confronting their own loss of life. She described how patients who were given a life-threatening diagnosis, like cancer, appeared to pass through four stages – denial (not me), anger, bargaining (for more time) and depression – before reaching psychological acceptance of death. The model is popular with nurses and other caring professions because they frequently encounter these types of reaction. The Kübler-Ross stages provide a framework for understanding aspects of adjustment to loss, but there is no evidence that people go through a series of invariant stages. Reactions to loss are very variable and it is often unhelpful to categorize dying people in terms of stages.

Parkes (1975) developed a model of bereavement loss based on clinical observations of those who had experienced major losses. He suggested that all significant losses result in a major and rapid change to people's taken-for-granted world (their schemas), which is threatening and frightening. He noted a number of common responses, many of which are similar to those noted by Kübler-Ross. The following list of grief reactions is drawn from observations of Kübler-Ross, Parkes, and Stroebe and Stroebe (1987):

Initial reactions
• Numbness, disbelief, unreality or denial
• Alarm reaction (see Chapter 7 on stress): experienced as anxiety, restlessness and fear

Common emotional and psychosocial responses
• Feelings of failure, regret or guilt
• Yearning and pining for the lost one
• Continuing to interact with the deceased, for example, feeling their presence and talking to them as though they were still there
• Feeling alone or abandoned
• Anger
• Sorrow, despair, pessimism, rumination
• Loss of purpose, feelings of loss of the self, loss of enjoyment, sense of worthlessness
• Difficulty in maintaining social relationships

Physical symptoms
• Insomnia
• Feelings of fatigue, lethargy, reduction in activity
• Slowed thinking, poor concentration
• Loss of appetite.

Wortman and Silver (1989) challenged some common assumptions made about bereavement loss:

• Is distress or depression inevitable? Studies of bereaved people show that not everyone becomes depressed. Research with widows conducted by Vachon *et al.* (1982) indicated that those who were most depressed in the early stages were also those most likely to be still depressed after two years.
• Is it important to 'work through' feelings of loss? It is assumed that resolution of grief requires cognitive-emotional processing and this is the aim

of interventions like psychotherapy or bereavement counselling. Yet studies suggest that people who exhibit high levels of yearning or pining tend to have a poorer outcome in the long term, regardless of intervention.

- Do all people resolve their grief? Models of loss assume that the final outcome of grieving will be a return to a normal psychological state. But Wortman and Silver (1989) suggested that for a minority of individuals grieving may continue over many years without necessarily being abnormal. It is difficult to know how long a 'normal' period of grieving lasts. It seems that sudden deaths such as in road traffic accidents, untimely deaths such those that involve children or young people, and those where there is no body are very difficult for bereaved people to come to terms with.

It might be assumed that the stronger the marital relationship, the greater the sense of loss when the partner dies. But Van Doorn *et al.* (1998) found that those who had had insecure attachment or dependent relationships were more likely to experience traumatic grief following the death of their spouse.

> Ted was devastated when Laura died. They had known each other since school, and had recently celebrated their golden wedding anniversary. She died of cancer after a relatively short illness, and Ted was quite unprepared for this. It was clear that he would find it difficult to look after himself because Laura had done all the housework, but he refused help. He could not bear the thought of leaving the house or of anyone else touching Laura's things. He sought refuge in his greenhouse and in the evenings felt Laura's presence by having all of her things around him. The family were concerned, but he refused all offers of help. Eventually, he developed bronchitis and moved in with Mark and Janice on a temporary basis. When he felt better, he visited his home and was able, with help, to clear a few things out. He now felt able to start letting go.

Grief can be seen to have many components and is best thought of as a holistic response to loss. Grief is a normal process, not a state, and does not involve a series of stages. Grief is painful and affects almost all aspects of the person. Many people describe grief as physically painful and may need reassurance that they are not ill. Some people may cope with their grief by increasing their use of mood-altering substances like alcohol, tobacco or drugs. These impede successful adaptation and contribute an added risk to health. It is known that there is an increased risk of death in the first few years after the death of a spouse. Loss leads to immunological suppression and increased susceptibility to infections and stress-related diseases (Chapter 7). Depression following bereavement leads to increased risk of suicide.

> Some time after the death of her father, a young woman returned to the
> hospital ward on which he died to thank the nursing staff. She explained
> that, despite the distress and pain she experienced when informed of her
> father's terminal condition and his subsequent death, she was grateful for
> the time period between these two events. Amongst other things, it gave
> her time to resolve conflicts, express her love and say goodbye.
>
> (Evans 1994: 160)

This extract suggests that we are able to help people prepare for a
bereavement and start to mourn their loss before death actually occurs.
Much of the care offered to relatives of dying patients is based on the
assumption that 'grief work' can begin prior to the death. It may help relatives to realistically face up to their imminent loss. The grief experienced at
that time will help prevent subsequent abnormal bereavement. However,
the research evidence about anticipatory grief is rather confused. Evans
(1994) suggested that instead of focusing just on the death, we should be
aware of the multiple stresses and losses that occur for patients and their
carers during a terminal illness and support them while they deal with
these.

Alzheimer's disease illustrates the protracted losses that can face a spouse
before the death of a loved one. For example, loss of the person they married and loved, the friend, social companion, lover, income provider, car
driver, person to argue with, and so on. These losses may occur gradually
over many years, each loss to be mourned and require adjustment. Very
extended periods of anticipatory grief may not be helpful, as 'grief work'
may involve emotional withdrawal from the loved person. Such a process
may not be adaptive for the carer of a person with a chronic illness because
their loved one still requires care. In addition, a withdrawal of emotional
involvement can induce a sense of guilt after the death has occurred.

Recent perspectives of loss and grief

Stroebe and Schut (1998) proposed a 'dual process' model of grief,
illustrated in Figure 5.1. Instead of proposing a linear trajectory towards
resolution, this identifies a process of oscillation between the feelings of grief,
and thoughts, feelings and behaviours directed towards restoration. Over
time, grief experiences diminish while restoration activities increase. Restoration experiences include doing new things, finding sources of distraction
and eventually finding new roles, identities and relationships. The rate at
which this occurs is very variable. Some people orient themselves towards
restoration at an early stage, such as undertaking activities in memory of
the person who has died. Examples include fund-raising in aid of a charity
associated with the illness experienced by the person who died, or involvement in a self-help group for those who have experienced similar losses.

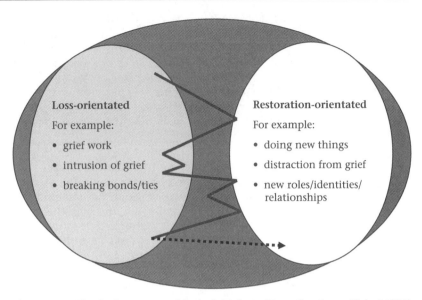

Figure 5.1 The dual process model of grief (adapted from Stroebe and Schut 1998).

But some people remain focused on loss. Those who engage in excessive rumination about their loss, long after the event, usually require professional help.

A 'biographical' perspective on loss was put forward by Walter (1996). Walter applied this to all forms of loss, including changes in body image. His theory proposed that a person who has experienced an important change or loss needs to construct or reconstruct their identity in the light of the changes that have occurred. This reflects a growing interest in **narrative psychology** (Chapter 2). Gergen and Gergen (1997), leading proponents of narrative psychology, identified that most people have a personal story that has a trajectory towards a desired goal. Our biography is what links our past with our present and our expectations for the future and gives a sense of coherence. Bury (1982) introduced the concept of biographical disruption to explain the impact of losses. This means that many of the taken-for-granted aspects of daily life and future expectations are disrupted and the notion of 'self' has to alter to accommodate these changes. Borrowing the notion of schemas, some people are able to accommodate change within their existing schemas, while others cannot.

Qualitative research often encourages story-telling. This can have therapeutic value as well as providing useful insights into the lived experience of common medical conditions.

Asbring (2001) interviewed women with fibromyalgia to find out how their illness had affected their sense of identity. Fibromyalgia is a painful condition that affects the muscles and for which there is no known effective treatment. Most of the interviewees were unable to continue

working, and one participant described her life as similar to that of a
pensioner. The main finding was that the illness led to a radical disruption
in the women's biographies and had a profound effect on their sense of
identity, particularly in relation to work and social life. However, not all of
the changes were negative, and many of the women also experienced
gains as a result of their illness. For example, they felt they had learned to
place more value on small joys and less on material goods.

It is important to come to terms with losses and integrate them into
continuing life, or mental health may suffer. According to Walter, story-
telling is the means by which people have traditionally achieved this. Kelly
(1998) described how coming to terms with the changes brought about by
these losses required what she termed 're-storying one's life'. The process
may reflect the psychological tasks to which Erikson (1980) referred. It
involves finding new goals and a new sense of purpose to one's life and
requires the individual to construct a new and different ongoing life story.
Narrative psychologists (Crossley 2003) and gerontologists (Clark 2001)
suggest that therapeutic work involves 'emplotment', through which
chaotic and disruptive memories are structured into a coherent and
meaningful story or plot. This is termed **narrative therapy**.

Conversations with friends, non-directive counselling, narrative writing
(see Chapter 7) and life review all provide opportunities for narrative therapy. This indicates that the most important task of the health professional,
when faced with someone who is bereaved, is to listen.

Walter published this quotation from an anonymous source. We have
reproduced it in poetic form to capture its full impact.

I am a student nurse. I am dying.
I write this to you who are, and will become, nurses
in the hope that by my sharing my feelings with you,
you may someday be better able to help those who share my experience.
For me, fear is today and dying is now.
You slip in and out of my room,
give me medications and check my blood pressure.
Is it because I am a student nurse myself, or just a human being,
that I sense your fright?
And your fears enhance mine.
Why are you afraid? I am the one who is dying. . . .
If only we could be honest, both admit our fear, touch one another.
If you really care,
would you lose so much of our valuable professionalism
if you even cried with me?. . .
Then it might not be so hard to die –
in a hospital – with friends close by.

(Walter 1996: 26)

Hope

Perhaps one of the reasons why many health care professionals find it so hard to confront death is because of our desire to maintain hope. This chapter ends where it started, with new beginnings and ways of seeing the world. Hope is what most of us live for. Snyder (1998) presented a theory of hope in situations involving pain, loss and suffering. He defined hope as a combination of a determination to achieve a desired goal or end point and a plan for getting there. When pain, illness, disability or any loss occurs, previously valued goals may be or seem unattainable. This can engender hopelessness, bring acceptance or promote determination.

A feature of those who maintain high hope is the ability to modify or change some of their original goals. This requires a willingness to change one's personal biography. Snyder identified that high-hope people have different goals within different life arenas. This means that they are able to switch to another goal when one appears unobtainable. He argued that grieving occurs when a previously attainable goal is no longer obtainable. However, following a period of mourning, high-hope people turn their attentions to substitute goals that are achievable. Health care professionals can help patients to face things one step at a time when faced with overwhelming challenges.

Early in her third year of training, Anna was placed in a hospice for people with all kinds of terminal illness. She was very anxious because she did not really know how to talk to people who were dying or how to approach other patients following a death. However, once she had started on the ward her mentor carefully discussed with her the philosophy of hospice care, the holistic approach and the emphasis on openness and sharing with patient, family and staff. The mentor helped Anna to understand her own reactions to death and dying. This enabled Anna to communicate in a positive way with others who were exploring their own issues in relation to dying. Anna was surprised to discover that, rather than being a place of sadness, there was a real sense of hope which focused on maximizing quality of life for the patients and their families.

Summary of key points

- Stage models of cognitive development offer some guidance to children's understandings at different ages, but there are wide individual variations and misconceptions are common.
- It is necessary to find out about a child's existing understanding of health and illness so that it is possible to help build on and extend this through demonstration and play, and not just talking.

- Secure attachment relationships, that involve parental warmth, involvement and monitoring, are important for normal psychological development and reduction of risk behaviours.
- When considering development across the lifespan, it is helpful to consider common challenges and demands within their ecological and cultural context, using a framework of stress and coping.
- It is important to recognize common responses to loss, but it is not helpful to conceptualize these as a series of inevitable stages.
- Narrative therapies help to maintain or restore a sense of coherence, particularly towards the end of life.
- Understanding the lived experience and listening to patients' stories has therapeutic value.
- Hope can be maintained by focusing on what is possible, rather than what is not.

Recommended reading

Cassidy, J. and Shaver, P.R. (eds) (1999) *Handbook of Attachment: Theory, Research and Clinical Applications*. New York: Guilford Press

Crossley, M.L. (2000) *Introducing Narrative Psychology: Self, Trauma and the Construction of Meaning*. Buckingham: Open University Press.

Harvey, J.H. (ed.) (1998) *Perspectives on Loss: A sourcebook*. Philadelphia: Brunner Maazel.

Walter, T. (1996) *The Revival of Death*. London: Routledge

CHAPTER SIX

SOCIAL PROCESSES IN HEALTH CARE

- What special techniques can be used to persuade people to change their beliefs and motivate them to want to change their behaviour?
- To what extent are we influenced by others when making important decisions, and what are the implications of this in health care?
- Why are some people more likely to receive help than others?
- What is non-verbal behaviour and why is it important in communication?
- How do groups influence decisions and behaviour, and what are the implications of this for interprofessional working?
- What is the best way to deal with complaints and conflict?

Introduction

In this chapter, we explore important social processes involved in interactions between professionals and patients and their families, between different groups of professionals, and between managers and workforce. The chapter is informed by research from social psychology. We commence by reviewing theories of persuasion that inform much of health and education activities. We then focus on social influences on behaviour within group or organizational settings. Much of western psychology concentrates exclusively on individual psychological processes such as memory, learning and aspects of self. Yet humans are social animals, and these processes are strongly influenced by those around us. To explore such issues, we have often integrated information from a variety of classic, original and secondary sources (e.g. Brehm *et al.* 2002) and this is why not every detail is referenced. We illustrate social influences with a selection of classic experiments from social psychology. We examine the lessons these hold for everyone working in the field of health care.

Persuasion

Persuasion is central to the implementation of many health promotion and education activities. Therefore it is useful to know some of the principles that can be used to enhance persuasion. These are also principles that are used in marketing and sales. Whether or not health should be marketed or sold in the same way poses interesting professional, moral and ethical issues. Nevertheless, research in public health has identified aspects of lifestyle that are known to affect mortality (death) and morbidity (illness) in the longer term. Examples of lifestyles associated with increased length and quality of life include taking regular exercise, not smoking, moderating alcohol intake and having a balanced diet that includes plenty of fresh fruit and vegetables. An important question addressed in this chapter is how this knowledge can be conveyed in a form that people will believe and feel motivated to want to follow. The content of this chapter is based on an accumulation of research going back over many years and can be found in any textbook on social psychology.

There are several basic steps in the persuasion process. First it is necessary to identify the target audience and customize the message to their particular needs. In order for the message to be assimilated, the audience must:

- see or hear the message. The sender must select a medium (television channel, radio network, newspaper or magazine, circulation of leaflets, etc.) that is likely to ensure that all of the target audience has easy access to it. Placing leaflets in a doctor's surgery, while cheap and convenient, is rarely an effective way to achieve this.
- pay attention to the message. Attention is selective, so the format of the message must be eye-catching. Presenting health information in a leaflet that does not immediately appeal to the target audience will ensure that people do not pick it up and read it. The audience must also see the message as relevant to them. For example, a PhD student studying osteoporosis in men found that the leaflets on osteoporosis contained only pictures of women, indicating that it is not a male issue (which is not true).
- understand the message. Hearing advice or reading information does not mean that everyone will be able to understand it (Chapter 3). It is the responsibility of health professionals to ensure that all people are able to understand the information given. This can be achieved by working with patient representatives when preparing it.
- accept the conclusion of the message. This is less likely if it conflicts with long-standing beliefs, or messages from other sources. For example, dietary information has been subject to periodic changes, leaving the public perplexed and sceptical.

Having understood the message, social psychologists have identified that acceptance is influenced by factors related to features of the sender, the message and the recipient.

The source or sender of the message

Several factors have been identified as influencing the recipient's judgement about the source or sender.

- Credibility. This does not always equate with knowledge of the topic. For example, nutritionists know most about diet, and physiotherapists about exercise, but the public may nevertheless see the doctor as a more credible source of information on these topics.

- Trustworthiness. Does the sender have anything to gain by persuading others? Health professionals are often seen as having a vested interest in health promotion. Evidence from social psychology suggests that messages may be more persuasive if the sender argues from a position that is apparently opposed to his or her self-interest. It could therefore be argued that a heavy drinker will take more notice of advice to cut down from a former alcoholic or heavy drinker rather than a health professional who does not drink.

- Attractiveness. People may view the sender as a role model for the lifestyle being promoted and reject the message if they see them as unattractive. It appears that the attractiveness of the communicator is more influential for relatively trivial messages than for serious ones. Nevertheless, health promoters may wish to pay attention to their personal appearance if they wish others to take note of them.

Petty and Cacioppo (1986) identified two distinct routes to persuasion. These involve an interaction between the source, the message and the audience. Those who are well educated and think carefully about health issues are more likely to focus on the significance and content of the message. Those who are less well educated and motivated are more likely to be persuaded by superficial images such as the attractiveness of the presenter or the advertisement (see Figure 6.1).

The nature of the message

Reason versus emotion

Many health promotion campaigns are designed to scare recipients into taking health action. A meta-analysis by Witte and Allen (2000) indicated that high-fear appeals are effective only if the recipient is confident that they are able to achieve the behaviour change recommended. In those who are not confident of being able to take prevention action, high-fear appeals result in avoidance rather than behaviour change. Messages must therefore be accompanied by clearly specified advice about simple and effective courses of action.

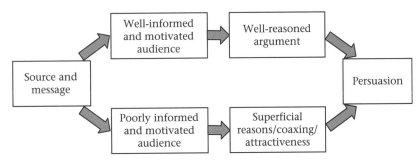

Figure 6.1 Dual process model of persuasion (based on Petty and Cacioppo 1986).

Humans have a strong tendency to focus upon individual situations that have strong emotional appeal, rather than on statistical or epidemiological evidence which has strong rational appeal. This is why many campaigns feature people with whom the target group are likely to identify. Television is the best medium for making emotional appeals since emotional images are stronger when they combine sight, sound and movement.

When trying to appeal to reason in order to convey a serious issue, it is worth considering if both sides of the argument should be presented. A well-informed audience is more likely to be persuaded by two-sided arguments because they will be aware of the counter-arguments and will wish to see these addressed. A less well-informed audience is likely to be confused by two-sided arguments and it may be better to present them with a single point of view.

Before Mark was diagnosed as having diabetes and hypertension, Janice knew that he was in a high-risk group because of his weight gain and high sugar intake. She warned him of the possible consequences if he carried on as he was, but he closed his ears, reasoning that nobody in his family had diabetes or heart problems and these were unlikely to happen to him. He was eventually persuaded by the diabetic consultant and nutritionist because they took the time to explain his condition to him and discuss the pros and cons of dietary and other lifestyle change.

Order of presentation

The importance of primacy and recency effects has already been discussed (Chapter 3). When presenting verbal arguments, health professionals often unwittingly influence clients' decisions by the order in which the issues are presented.

Cognitive dissonance

Leon Festinger observed that when an individual holds two or more beliefs that are inconsistent with each other, they experience a state of dissonance. For example, 'I am a healthy person' may conflict with the knowledge that 'I do not take enough exercise'. Therefore, when individuals are presented with health messages that conflict with their current behaviour, this creates a sense of cognitive dissonance. According to his theory of cognitive dissonance (Festinger 1957), this state of dissonance is unsettling and needs to be resolved. This involves either modifying or justifying their behaviour.

Aronson (1988) suggested that alternatives for those confronted with discrepant messages are to:

- change their opinion;
- induce the communicator to change his or her opinion;
- seek support for their original opinion from supporters;

- convince themselves that the communicator is untrustworthy or uncreditworthy.

It has been found that the greater the discrepancy between the argument being presented and the individual's current attitudes, the less the extent of attitude change (this fits with the concept of the mental **schema**; see Chapters 3 and 5). Therefore it is important to find out about the current beliefs of the target or audience and try to work out a solution that they can accommodate.

Mark had originally closed his ears to health messages because they contradicted a lifestyle that he enjoyed, notably eating crisps and chocolate and drinking beer. He thought that dietary advice was just a fad and 'they' would think of something else next week. When Janice tried to persuade him to change, he reasoned that she was not an expert on diet and sought support from his friends in the pub.

Complexity and presentation of the message

Complex information cannot be assimilated quickly and requires repetition. Therefore, where complex information is given to patients, it should be provided in written (or possibly taped) format so that they can take it away and study it at their leisure.

When Sasha attended her first antenatal check, when she was expecting Lee, she was asked if she wished to have a screening test for congenital abnormalities in her unborn child. Although the midwife explained the tests carefully, Anna had difficulty understanding the full implications. The choices she was asked to make were also complex. If she had the screening done, what were the options if the tests were positive? If she chose not to the have the screening done, what were the potential consequences for her and her family? She agreed to the tests because she did not want to waste the midwife's time or appear foolish. But she was quite uncertain about the answers to these questions. When she became pregnant this time, she made sure that she had read and understood the leaflets she was given at the doctor's surgery. She discussed them with Janice and with Jo before her first hospital antenatal check. This time she felt more confident and was able to ask questions to assure herself that she was making the right decision.

Immediacy of action and endurance of the message

Health promoting messages quickly lose their effect. The longer the gap between receiving the persuasive message and taking health-protective action, the more likely it is that other factors will intervene, and the more likely it is that the individual will find justifications and counter-arguments. Therefore, it is helpful if individuals are persuaded to make an immediate act of commitment, much in the same way that religious evangelists invite audience members to make an immediate declaration of commitment. This is why the salesman tries hard to make an immediate sale. Psychologists sometimes use contracts to confirm their client's commitment to an agreed behaviour change.

Once initiated, the new attitude must be sustained in order to preserve the behaviour change. Therefore, health promotion is more likely to be effective if the message or media image is maintained in the public domain over a long period of time. Mass campaigns are largely ineffectual unless the impetus is maintained.

When Mark was seen by the nutritionist, they reviewed his current diet and made a plan of change that would be achievable. He was asked to record his eating pattern and to see the diabetic nurse for a review. This made it more difficult for him to go home and forget or ignore what he had been told, or be tempted to cheat too drastically.

Audience influences and effects

Selective attention

It is well recognized that people tend to focus attention on issues that reflect their existing understanding or point of view. This again reflects the concept of the mental schema (Chapters 3 and 5).

In an old but relevant study, Kleinhesselink and Edwards (1975) asked university students to complete a questionnaire concerning their attitudes to the legalization of cannabis. They then listened to a broadcast, through headphones, that contained seven strong (irrefutable) arguments and seven weak (refutable) arguments in favour of legalization. Constant static noise made listening difficult, but students could press a button to reduce this. Those who favoured legalization pushed the button significantly more often when strong arguments were presented. Subjects who opposed legalization pushed the button significantly more often

> when weak (refutable) arguments were presented. The conclusion of this study was that individuals pay more attention to messages that support their own beliefs.

Festinger (1954) formulated social comparison theory, which proposed that individuals deliberately seek validation of their own attitudes and beliefs by attending to those who hold ideas similar to their own, and distancing themselves from those who hold different beliefs or attitudes. This means that some social groups, such as teenagers, may be difficult to penetrate by those seen as outsiders. Health educators need to find novel ways of gaining acceptance if health messages are to be received and taken seriously.

> When Jo left school, he regularly took drugs, including alcohol and ecstasy, as did all his friends. Janice tried to warn him that this was not a good idea, but this simply drove him out of the house to meet his mates, thus reinforcing his attitudes. When he met Sasha, he spent less time with these friends and started using alcohol and drugs less frequently.

Self-esteem and compliance

People with low **self-esteem** do not place high value on their own ideas and are therefore more likely to be compliant. They may also be more likely to give in to peer pressure if this conflicts with advice from health professionals. People with high self-esteem are more likely to question and challenge, but may be persuaded by rational argument. Education provides people with essential knowledge and life skills and is an important source of **self-efficacy** and self-esteem.

In summary

Health-promoting messages need to be tailored to the needs of the audience. Those who are well educated, well motivated and have high self-esteem are more likely to respond to full information and a well reasoned argument from a credible source. These may be future trend-setters and are therefore an important target audience for health promotion. Those who are less well educated and have low self-esteem are more likely to respond to superficial but directive messages from attractive and emotionally appealing sources with whom they are able to identify. Health messages that contradict prevailing social and cultural beliefs and behaviours, particularly those within cohesive subcultures, are likely to be resisted. These issues are best addressed by group members working from within.

Obedience to authority

Persuasion appeals to reason, whereas obedience does not. Obedience means 'do as you are told without asking questions'. Stanley Milgram was a psychologist at Yale University in the 1960s who was interested in understanding how Hitler was able to induce mass obedience to engage in extreme acts of cruelty during the Second World War. He set up a famous laboratory experiment that turned out to have implications far beyond his expectations.

Milgram advertised for volunteers to take part in an educational experiment at Harvard University. On arrival, each volunteer was introduced to another participant and a draw took place to identify who would be the pupil and who the teacher in the experiment. In fact, the draw was fixed and the volunteer always took the part of the teacher. The 'teacher' was told by the experimenter to press a button to give the 'pupil' an electric shock as a punishment if he made a mistake. The shocks gradually increased in intensity from 15 volts to 450 volts, the upper range clearly marked on the dial in red as 'danger'.

It came as a shock to all concerned that 26 out of the 40 subjects continued, on instruction from the experimenter, to give up to 450 volts of shock even though the pupil had progressed through protests and screams and was by this time looking as though they might be unconscious. Nobody stopped at below 300 volts (the British household voltage is 240 volts and the American voltage 110 volts).

The following features have subsequently been shown to influence obedience in this type of experimental situation:

- The legitimacy or status of the authority figure. When the experiment was repeated at a less well-known institution, obedience was less likely, although still occurred at an alarming level.
- The proximity of victim. Obedience was less likely when the victim was in the same room, rather than behind a glass screen.
- The proximity of the authority figure. Obedience was less likely when the experimenter was in another room and gave instructions by telephone.
- Personal characteristics. Some volunteers appeared to be more conformist than others and less obedient to instruction.
- Habit. Some people appeared to respond automatically to authority cues.
- Social rules of commitment. Having agreed to participate in the experiment, the volunteers felt obliged to do as they were asked.

Does obedience to authority happen in health care?

A 'real-life' experiment was conducted by Hofling *et al.* (1966). A drug marked 'Astroten 5 mg, maximum dose 10 mg' was planted in the drugs cabinet on a mental health care ward. The experimenter, purporting to be a psychiatrist, phoned the ward and asked the nurse in charge to give a named patient 20 mg of Astroten. An observer intercepted the nurse before she (they were all female) reached the patient. All except one of the 22 nurses complied with the instruction even though:

- there was no written prescription;
- the drug exceeded the safe dose (11 claimed not to have noticed this);
- none of the nurses had ever heard of either the drug or the 'doctor' beforehand.

Could this type of problem occur today?

Anna had recently qualified and was working on a unit that undertook invasive investigations for which there is a long waiting list. The procedure required the routine administration of a drug one hour beforehand. The drug was harmless in the dose normally given, but could be harmful in higher doses. The Trust rules stated that she was not allowed to give a drug without a doctor's written prescription. On this occasion, a new registrar whom she had not yet met had forgotten to write up the drug for one of the patients who had been waiting for half an hour. He phoned to inform Anna that he was otherwise engaged. He was very nice and apologetic. He asked Anna to administer the drug and he would sign for it as soon as he could get away. What should Anna do? What if the patient was a well known figure likely to cause a scene at being kept waiting? What if the registrar expresses apprehension about the consultant's reaction to his mistake?

One of the main reasons for introducing diploma- or degree-level training for all health care professionals is to raise awareness of these issues, encourage questioning and consider the potential consequences before accepting or giving orders.

Conformity

In the section on persuasion, we mentioned the importance of peer group pressure. The tendency to conform with the beliefs and behaviours of others is an important source of social influence, and **social norms** form a component of social cognitive theories, used to predict health behaviour (Chapter 8). Conformity, like obedience, has been shown to affect our behaviour in ways that can have serious implications for health care provision.

Conformity was demonstrated in a classic psychology experiment by Solomon Asch in the early 1950s. Male college students volunteered to take part in an experiment that they were told involved visual judgement. They were shown a line on a card and asked to match it with the length of one of three lines shown on a separate card (as shown in Figure 6.2). This is an extremely straightforward and unambiguous task. However, each student was unknowingly placed in a room with confederates of the experimenter who deliberately selected the wrong line. In this situation, one third of students gave the same 'wrong' answer as the one given by the confederates. Seventy per cent of students conformed on at least one occasion. Only a minority remained independent in the face of this type of group pressure.

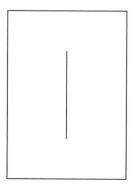 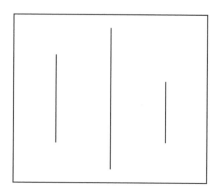

Figure 6.2   Presentation similar to that used in the Asch experiment on conformity. Participants were asked to match the length of the line on the left-hand card with one of the lines on the right-hand card.

It appears that people are prepared to deny the evidence of their own senses if this is contradicted by the beliefs or behaviour of others.

Imagine you are a student nurse, like Anna, working on a first clinical placement. You are asked to take a routine blood pressure. You are not confident and are unable to detect meaningful sounds at the first attempt. What are you likely to do? You try again, and this time you are reasonably confident with the result. However, it is much lower than the patient's previous recordings. What do you do? The pressure is checked by another nurse who, having first checked the chart, confidently announces a pressure in line with previous recordings. You try again and obtain the same lower recording. How do you feel? What do you do?

Conformity to the views and behaviour of other people has been shown to be more likely in certain circumstances:

• When the task is difficult or the information available is ambiguous or sparse. This is true of many situations in health care.
• When the desire for social approval overrides other aspects of judgement.
• When contradicting the judgement of someone else might appear rude or discourteous.
• If the others are perceived to have a greater level of expertise. Novices may be correct, but it is the views of experts which are generally heeded.
• If the confidence, self-esteem and self-efficacy of the individual is low.

These conditions commonly apply in health care. They explain why patients are reluctant to question or disagree with the advice they are given. They explain why patients give consent to procedures even when they have not understood what they have been told. They explain why nurses may sometimes fail to question instructions.

It often takes considerable courage to stand up for one's convictions or question authority. Brehm *et al.* (2002) suggested that people are less likely to conform in individualistic societies that value self-reliance and more likely to conform in collectivist societies that value cooperation and family and social allegiances. However, in individualistic societies, adolescents tend to form groups or gangs to assert their individualism. Adherence to these **reference group** norms is very strong. Non-conformity and non-compliance are higher among those with a strong desire for self-expression. But this is often regarded by others as evidence of deviance, eccentricity, or 'being difficult'.

The failure of individuals to act on their own beliefs can have important consequences in organizational settings. James Reason (1990) undertook an analysis of a number of major disasters and identified that this was a significant contributory factor. In the case of the Chernobyl disaster, the local maintenance team appear to have assumed that a team of experts from Moscow knew what they were doing and were in control of the situation, even though they could see that the dials clearly registered danger levels. The hierarchical organization of the National Health Service encourages obedience and compliance and is vulnerable to this type of mistake.

Anna started work on a busy surgical ward and observed that the nursing staff were not applying sterile dressings in accordance with hospital policy, as she had been taught. She recognized that this could have serious consequences for patients and drew this to the attention of the staff nurse. The nurse became quite angry and told her that there was no time to be fussy on this ward. Anna was faced with the choice of either being labelled 'difficult' or conforming with poor practice. What would you do in these circumstances?

It often takes a serious incident to draw attention to these types of practice, even though there is clearly an accident waiting to happen. It is difficult to deal with these types of situation alone, since 'whistleblowers' are often discredited (see also Chapter 2 on stigma). Ideally it is best to gain support from others, though this may be difficult.

Social desirability

Social desirability refers to the tendency to answer questions in a socially approved manner. Many people are willing to lie in order to put forward a good impression of themselves. This is an important reason why patients do not always tell the truth about their lifestyle or taking of medications. It is also an important consideration for those undertaking research in health care that relies on self-report. Individuals invariably try to interpret what is required of them and may modify their responses as part of their own impression management (Chapter 2). This is why social researchers frequently have to use false cover stories.

In social survey research, researchers sometimes use the Crowne–Marlowe Social Desirability Scale (Crowne and Marlowe 1960) to identify those whose responses are strongly influenced by the wish to portray themselves in a positive light. An example from the scale includes the item: 'When I hear people talking privately I avoid listening'. It is assumed that all of us have listened in on a private conversation at some time. Therefore, those answering no to this and a series of similar questions are judged to demonstrate social desirability bias. This is why, in clinical practice, it is important to ask open questions to elicit people's own views or understanding, rather than asking questions that require a yes/no answer. For example, when 'consenting' someone, it is desirable to ask what they have understood about what is going to happen. This approach to questioning gives less opportunity for conformity and compliance.

Helping others

This book is written for those working or training to work in the caring professions. But what is it that drives people to want to help others? Do some professionals help only because they are paid to do so? What motivates people to volunteer to help others?

There are some intrinsic rewards to be gained from helping others. Helping others may elicit social approval or praise and makes people feel good. Another explanation involves reciprocal altruism. This reflects the belief that if I help someone else, they may help me if or when I need it. This applies to groups as well as to individuals. Self-help groups are often set up by people who have received help and wish to share their knowledge and experience.

Omoto and Snyder (1995) identified five reasons why people volunteered to work with AIDS patients.

- Humanitarian values: wanting to help others; being a caring person.
- Curiosity: the desire to learn more about illness or disability and to reduce personal fears and anxieties.
- Personal and social development: meeting new people, making new friends; gaining experience of dealing with difficult topics.
- Social obligation: concern for a particular underprivileged group in society.
- Esteem/control enhancement: to feel good, escape from other pressures, feel less lonely.

Most health professionals, if we are honest, will admit to coming into the profession for at least three of these reasons, quite apart from the issues of pay and career prospects.

Janice became a health care assistant after her children had gone to school because she needed something to do and wanted to get out of the house to meet new people. She was interested in helping others, particularly older people. But she was also curious to learn more about the treatment of various diseases and disorders that she had heard of, but knew little about.

The next subsection considers the issue of helping in situations that involve strangers and where the motivations to assist appear less strong.

Taking responsibility in an emergency

Social psychologists became interested in studying the phenomenon of bystander apathy following an incident in the USA when a young woman, Kitty Genovese, was brutally murdered outside a block of flats. Her cries for help over a half-hour period were heard by a large number of people, yet no one phoned for the police, and the report of this shocked the nation.

Latané and Darley (1968) subsequently staged a series of 'emergencies' to explore the circumstances in which bystanders were more or less likely to intervene. A typical situation involved a man collapsed on an underground train. They identified quite a few factors likely to be influential in determining helping action.

- People are more likely to act if there are cues to the seriousness of the situation from other bystanders. Once one person initiates action, others will follow.

- The larger the number of strangers present who do nothing, the less likely an individual is to intervene. Each individual assumes that someone else will take the necessary action.
- People fail to act if they perceive themselves as incapable of doing anything to help. Conversely, they are more likely to act if they feel they can do something useful to help.
- People are less likely to act in ambiguous situations. For example, people may ignore someone lying on the pavement in the expectation that they are drunk, rather than ill.
- People are more likely to take action if they have the opportunity to discuss the situation with other people first.
- Helping actions are influenced by the perceived 'deservedness' or culpability of the victim. This may relate to a 'just world' hypothesis in which people are presumed to get what they deserve in life.
- The extent to which the 'victim' is perceived to be attractive. People who are facially, physically or behaviourally unattractive are less likely to receive sympathy or help.
- People are more likely to help if they are in a good mood!

Health care professionals are all trained to administer basic life support and are probably more likely to help in emergency situations. Therefore, it is helpful to be aware that once you have initiated action others are likely to follow and be supportive.

Non-verbal communication

Attitudes were described in Chapter 2 as evaluative responses, such as approval and disapproval. These are often expressed through non-verbal communication. If we disapprove of someone, or if we are nervous or annoyed, it is very hard to cover up these feelings. Studies of patient satisfaction with health care have repeatedly shown that interpersonal aspects of care are central to patients' perceptions of quality of care. It is not just what we do, as health professionals, it is the way that we do it that is important. We reveal a lot about ourselves through non-verbal communication. For example, we signal confidence or nervousness through our body posture, hand movements, facial expression, tone of voice and speed of delivery. Empathy, understanding, caring, pain and distress all involve communication, and non-verbal behaviours are the main ways of communicating caring.

Positive and negative attitudes such as pleasure or annoyance, approval or disgust, are revealed through non-verbal signals. Eye contact with a friendly smile normally conveys interest and a willingness to engage. People frequently use the avoidance of eye contact to signal that they have no wish to engage in social interaction. This may be why nurses become adept at walking through a ward without making eye contact. But while this prevents diversions, it can leave patients feeling ignored and frustrated. Non-friendly eye contact is seen in many cultures as a mark of disrespect or act of aggression. Brehm *et al.* (2002) reported that eye contact can provoke attack in an unfriendly encounter.

Managing conflict

Conflict is an inevitable consequence of life. It is caused by competition for scarce resources, competing ideologies, and stereotypes and prejudice. Conflict can easily progress from feelings of threat or annoyance to aggression and violence. Violence by patients or their caregivers against staff has increased in the National Health Service. It is important to recognize the potential of our own actions to cause aggression or violence in others and not just to place the blame on those who are unable to control their behaviour.

The most important way of avoiding conflict is to try to understand the perspective or point of view of the other party. If someone comes to a hospital or clinic, they are normally trying to communicate a need. When someone complains or gets annoyed it is usually because they feel that their needs have not been recognized or responded to in the way they feel appropriate.

The natural response to a complaint or criticism is to defend one's position and offer an explanation. But a defensive response is usually interpreted as counter-attack and serves to intensify feelings of annoyance. It is necessary first to listen to the individual and acknowledge their needs. An apology for any annoyance or distress caused to an individual is useful in building or maintaining good interpersonal relationships. Patient services managers have recently become rather good at using this approach to deal with patient complaints.

Janice, in her 'helping' role as health care assistant, gave a patient some advice. The staff nurse told Janice off because it was for trained staff to deal with this. Janice, believing that she was acting in the patient's best interest, responded defensively. This led to bad feeling between the two members of staff, each of whom saw themselves as the victim of the other's persecution.

This type of situation is easily resolved if one of the players stops defending their position and apologizes. The other, not wishing to be pushed into the role of persecutor by refusing to accept an apology, will normally respond in the role of rescuer by saying 'that's alright' or 'don't worry about it' or 'it wasn't really your fault'.

Janice acknowledged that she should have checked with the staff nurse and apologized. The staff nurse told Janice that she was only doing her best for the patient and to think no more about it.

Knowledge of these rules of engagement can help in all sorts of potentially confrontational situations. People with aggressive tendencies tend to expect and perceive hostility in others. When confronted with people who appear angry, remember to act as rescuer and not as victim:

1. Acknowledge, verbally, that you have seen that they are angry. Look concerned.
2. Ask them what they are angry about. Look interested.
3. Acknowledge their right to feel angry in the situation as they perceived it (this is not the same as admitting responsibility). Look sympathetic.
4. Try to negotiate a solution. Look sincere. The rules of reciprocity now oblige the angry party to listen to the reasons why you might have difficulty meeting their demands.

Rules of reciprocity and conventions of communication break down under the influence of alcohol or drugs, particularly when people are aroused because of fear or anxiety. People are disinhibited when drunk or driven by the need to fuel a drug addiction. In these situations, it is necessary to avoid any verbal or non-verbal behaviour, such as eye contact, that might be interpreted, rightly or otherwise, as unsympathetic or confrontational. Similarly, touch can provoke attack if seen as an attempt to dominate or control. Hence, those working in situations where there is a high risk of attack, such as mental health units or accident and emergency departments, should receive special training in conflict avoidance and management.

The importance of individualized care

Feeling valued is one of the key determinants of patient trust and satisfaction (Walker *et al.* 1998). The opposite of feeling valued is feeling depersonalized and alienated. Depersonalization means treating someone as an object rather than as a person. The medical model of care can encourage this by focusing attention on the disease or injury, or by emphasizing dispositional factors in accounting for people's responses to illness (Chapter 2). One of the main antidotes to depersonalization, discrimination and conflict in health care is individualized, client-centred care, which recognizes individual beliefs, expectations and needs during the assessment, planning and implementation of care strategies. Kleinman (1988) asserted that the ability to listen to and interpret people's experiences of illness should be seen as core skills for health care professionals. Another remedy is the use of a holistic assessment which takes into account the environmental and situational constraints and resources within which the individual patient is functioning.

The rewards of caring for older people become apparent once an individualized approach to care is adopted. Task-oriented care focuses mainly upon the rituals of toileting, bathing, changing and feeding, which can easily become demoralizing for carers and patients. In contrast, individualized care can elicit rich rewards by establishing relationships and revealing anecdotes and personal histories. The tasks become less onerous for the patient and the nurse as they engage in a closer rapport. Some tasks may become less necessary as the nurse and patient work together to identify reasons for particular behaviour patterns. But the maintenance of patient-centred care at a time of immense pressures on health services staff calls for strong leadership.

Psychological perspectives on leadership

Just as the rise of Hitler and the aftermath of Hitler's Germany stimulated Stanley Milgram's work on obedience, so it stimulated Kurt Lewin to study the issue of leadership. Lewin had escaped from Nazi Germany before the War and initiated a series of studies with colleagues in America into the effects of authoritarian, democratic and *laissez-faire* leadership styles. These styles of leadership are similar to the classification used to describe parenting styles (Chapter 5). These experiments revealed the following findings:

- Democratic leadership encourages participation, engenders a sense of ownership and commitment within the group and generally leads to higher morale, friendliness, cooperation and productivity.
- Authoritarian leadership is based upon coercion and is generally associated with lower morale among the group or workforce. It can be useful in order to achieve an important task quickly, but may place undue stress upon some members of the group.

Most people prefer to work under strong but democratic leadership. Although psychological research has focused upon personality characteristics of good leaders, leadership also involves skills and techniques that do not come automatically. Therefore, management training is essential in the preparation of those who are appointed to take on leadership roles within health services, particularly at a time of rapid change. One of the main challenges for health service leaders is to break down barriers between different professional groups and promote interprofessional working.

Groups and group interactions

Irving Janis, a psychologist famous for his work on stress, was prompted by a major international incident to investigate group decision-making in more depth. The incident was the American decision, in 1961, to support the unsuccessful invasion of Cuba in what became known as the 'Bay of Pigs' disaster. This prompted the Cuban missile crisis of 1962 and led the American president, Kennedy, to admit that a dreadful mistake had been made by his highly expert group of advisers. But how did this happen and why? Janis (1982) analysed the group processes involved and proposed that they had been victims of 'groupthink'. Some of the main symptoms of groupthink are identified below.

- Illusions of invulnerability. Positions of power can lead people to believe that they cannot be proved wrong.
- Collective rationalization. Unrealistic assessments are supported by 'rational' arguments and used to convince other group members.
- Belief in the inherent morality of the group. This reflects the belief that the group is in the right and good must triumph.
- Stereotypes of out-groups. Outsiders are often automatically classified as 'bad guys' or enemies who must therefore be in the wrong.
- Direct pressure on dissenters. Dissenters are silenced and this discourages critical evaluation. Certain group members may take the initiative to reduce dissent by persuasion or coercion, and foster an illusion of unanimity. Silence is interpreted as support.

Groupthink leads to biased and often wrong decisions that are not based on the best available evidence. It is wise to be aware of these effects as members of formal or informal social groupings, and particularly important when contributing to a formal team charged with a specific task. Work on group or team composition suggests that groups which include a mixture of individuals with different skills and viewpoints are probably more effective in reaching an informed decision. 'Heterogeneous' groups are less likely to succumb to groupthink. Group size is an important consideration. It is rare for groups exceeding 12 to be effective, while a group of 5 or 6 people facilitates the active participation of each member. The chairperson plays an important and impartial role in encouraging each member to voice their opinions, and encourage the debate of any doubts. These principles underpin developments in interprofessional learning and problem-based learning.

The potentially divisive nature of social groupings, in terms of intergroup discrimination and prejudice, was demonstrated by Tajfel (1982). Tajfel's work suggests that members of a social group generally work towards maximizing profits or rewards for members of their own group (the in-group), often at the expense of other groups (the out-group). Illustrations of this are to be found in the vigorous defence of pay differentials within industry and battles between specialties for scarce resources within health services. Within health care, examples of in-group–out-group conflict have been found in the relationships between different professional groups, hospital and community, private and public services, and similar units in different localities.

Anna had the opportunity to sit in on multiprofessional case conferences held regularly to plan treatment and care for patients in an elderly care unit. It soon became clear that the group was not operating effectively. For example, the consultant persistently arrived late, put forward his point of view, and then left. Another group member always selected a higher chair than the others and tried to direct decisions. Eventually, a senior nurse broached this with other individual group members and found that nobody was satisfied with the meetings or the quality of the decisions reached. Group members identified that the room was too small and the furniture was inappropriate to facilitate sharing; decisions were not fully agreed and as a consequence were not implemented. As a result of this investigation, a larger and more comfortable meeting room was found and a set of ground rules agreed, which stipulated how the meeting should be run. These included all professionals dedicating time to attend, having a rotating chairperson, a short presentation by the lead professional, limited time for discussion, and an agreed plan of action with named persons responsible for implementation.

Groups work better when working towards an agreed goal. Observations of meetings at various levels in health care suggest that group representatives are often good at voicing what they want to do, but not always clear about what they wish to achieve. This can sometimes lead to conflict or chaos, but often leads weaker contributors to give in to the ideas of strong members, regardless of their appropriateness. Sharing an agreed goal helps to keep group activity focused and reduces sources of disagreement, since it is easier to argue against activity that is not directed towards the achievement of the goal. Further discussion of goals in health care is included in Chapter 7.

Summary of key points

- Persuasion can be enhanced by paying attention to particular features of the message sender, the nature of the message, characteristics of the target audience and immediacy of action or commitment to action.
- Obedience to authority figures and the desire to conform may occur without awareness, and can easily lead to unprofessional, unethical or undesirable practice.
- Helping and caring attitudes and responses are more easily elicited by those who are judged attractive or deserving.
- Non-verbal behaviour is an important source of communication in health care.
- Complaints and conflict may be diffused by listening to, understanding, responding appropriately to and acknowledging the other person's point of view.
- The creation of homogeneous groups, strong group identities and poorly determined goals can lead to intergroup conflict, poor decisions and poor interprofessional working.

Further reading

Brehm, S.S., Kassin, S.M. and Fein S. (2002) *Social Psychology*, 5th edition. Boston: Houghton Mifflin.

STRESS AND COPING

KEY

QUESTIONS

- **What is meant by the term 'stress'?**
- **How can we understand stress and coping?**
- **What is the relationship between physiological and psychological responses to stress?**
- **Are there individual differences in responses to stress?**
- **What are the important characteristics of stressful situations?**
- **What do we mean by 'social support'?**
- **How does stress influence health and illness?**
- **How can health care professionals help themselves and others to deal with stress?**

Introduction

Many people suffer from stress these days. Briner (1994) argued that in the late twentieth century, stress had become a modern myth, similar to demons and witches in the Middle Ages or 'nerves' in the 1950s. So what exactly does 'stress' mean? There are many common symptoms that could be indicative of stress:

Emotional
- Feeling upset and crying more than usual
- Feeling irritable and behaving unreasonably
- Losing your sense of humour
- Unreasonable fears

Cognitive
- Feeling a failure
- Worrying a lot
- Difficulty in making decisions
- Not wanting to be bothered

Behavioural
- Not eating, or eating too much
- Taking time off for minor illnesses
- Using alcohol, tobacco or other substances
- Withdrawing from usual activities

Physiological
- Having difficulty sleeping
- Indigestion or nausea
- Panic attacks
- Headaches and muscle tension.

We all experience some of these symptoms some of the time, but may have a stress-related illness if we experience quite a lot of them most of the time. Stress can have important consequences for health professionals and patients. A difficult problem when caring for patients is that many of these symptoms are also symptomatic of mental illness or physical disease. For example, in patients it can worsen or mask symptoms of other illnesses, or give rise to behaviours that increase health risk. In staff, stress can lead to **burnout**. Therefore stress and coping are very important concepts in health care.

Definitions of stress

There many definitions of stress in the literature. This is because stress is not a fact, but a concept that depends on a theoretical explanation. One of the simplest and most commonly used definitions of stress reflects the notion of 'imbalance': 'Stress refers to an imbalance between a perceived demand and the perceived ability of the individual to respond to it' (McGrath, 1970).

Theories of stress assume that there is:

- a stressor that poses a demand, challenge or threat;
- an awareness or perception of the stressor;
- a response that includes emotional, cognitive, behavioural and physiological changes.

Some people find certain situations stressful because they are unfamiliar and they do not know how to respond. Others hardly notice the same situation because it is familiar and they respond automatically.

> When Anna started her degree course at university, she had little idea what was expected of her and felt very anxious. She envied third-year students who seemed so confident. At that stage, it would have been easy to give up and go and work in a shop. But she stayed and by her second year had a much better idea of what was expected. By this time, she was enjoying the challenges of nursing. The things that had bothered her so much in her first year no longer seemed so difficult, and she felt much more relaxed and confident.

Not all stressors are bad for us. The effort of addressing challenges boosts our self-esteem, our skills and our immune systems, and prepares us to deal with future challenges. But what is challenging for one person may be stressful for another. A psychological theory of stress must account for these differences in response, and this is addressed in the transactional model of stress and coping.

The transactional model of stress and coping

The transactional model of stress was proposed by Richard Lazarus in the 1960s and later developed with Susan Folkman into the best-known theory of stress and coping. Previous models had failed to explain why some individuals find a particular situation stressful and others not. For example, the behaviourist view assumed that there was a direct relationship between the situational demand (the stressor) and the emotional and behavioural stress response. But this is clearly not the case since different individuals respond differently to the same or similar demands. Using a psychodynamic framework, stress-related problems associated with anxiety and depression might be attributed to poor attachment relationships in early life (Chapter 5). But this fails to recognize the stress-provoking characteristics of certain situations. The Lazarus model is a social cognitive model that identifies cognitive appraisal as the mediator between the situational demand and the individual response. It is summarized in Figure 7.1, where we have also mapped out phases of physiological response (Selye 1956). The concepts shown in Figure 7.1 are all referred to in the following sections.

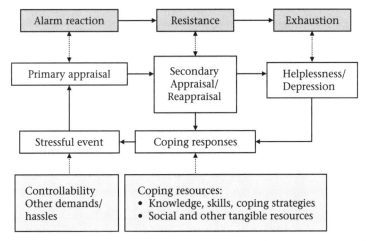

Figure 7.1 Overview of stress and coping processes (based on Lazarus and Folkman 1984; Seyle 1956).

Appraisal

Cognitive **appraisal** is part of the process of perception in which the individual determines if the situation poses a threat and decides what, if anything, to do about it. Appraisal is not necessarily a conscious process, since we respond automatically to a wide range of common situations. Differences in the ways that individuals interpret and respond to situations help to explain individual differences in response to similar demands.

> When people experience the same illness, they may react in quite different ways. One person may view the symptoms as unimportant. Another may view the symptoms as important but manageable. Yet another may view the same symptoms as catastrophic. Take the example of three people with back pain. The first person may have learned to get on with life and ignore the pain. The second may experience frequent pain, but has learned to manage it using a combination of prescribed medications, complementary therapies, gentle exercise and keeping busy. The third may find the pain completely unbearable and keep going to the doctor in the hope of finding a cure. Each of these three people may be described as having a different ways of appraising and coping with the pain.

Lazarus (1966) was the first theorist to identify thought processes as mediators between the situational demand (the stressor) and the emotional and behavioural coping response. Lazarus and Averill (1972: 243) proposed a three-stage model of appraisal.

- Primary appraisal is the immediate response to a new demand, situation or event when the individual determines if this represents a threat. There are three possible outcomes to primary appraisal: the situation is disregarded as irrelevant or unimportant; it is evaluated as a challenge likely to have a positive outcome if appropriate action is taken; or it is identified as a potential threat to physical or mental well-being.
- Secondary appraisal refers to the appraisal of coping alternatives, during which the individual decides what to do about the perceived threat. Very broadly, the behavioural choices available reflect the three dimensions of locus of control and include: taking personal action to deal with the situation (internal or personal control); seeking help from others to deal with the situation (External powerful other control); doing nothing or ignoring it (External chance control).
- Reappraisal then takes place. This is where the individual considers the appropriateness of their judgement and the outcome of their coping response.

The outcome of primary appraisal is largely determined by previous experiences. Those who have previously dealt successfully with similar demands are more likely to perceive a challenge than a threat. Those who have no experience of similar situations, and have little information about what is happening, are likely to experience uncertainty, anxiety or help-lessness. Those who have experienced difficulties or problems in similar previous situations are likely to perceive a threat and react with fear, anxiety or sense of hopelessness. This is why information and education are so important in all types of health care situation (Chapter 3).

Secondary appraisal and reappraisal are likely to be influenced by the individual's knowledge about the controllability of the situation, their beliefs about their ability (or that of others) to achieve a successful out-come (**locus of control**) and their sense of **self-efficacy** in using rele-vant practical and problem-solving skills. If the individual has not encountered similar situations before, they are less likely to experience stress if they have information about the best way to deal with the situ-ation or have help to achieve a successful outcome. Health care profes-sionals can do much to assist patients facing new or difficult situations by showing them the best ways to deal with it and supporting them until they feel confident.

> When Mark was admitted to hospital for the first time, he was very anxious because he did not know what to expect or what was expected of him. But he was given an information sheet telling him what he needed to take with him, what to expect, when visiting hours were, etc. This did much to reduce his stress and anxiety. The helpful manner in which he was greeted on the ward, shown round, introduced to other patients and informed about what would happen next was very reassuring.

Demographic influences on appraisal and coping

Those who lack knowledge, skills and experience are clearly disadvantaged when faced with new demands. This explains why stress responses may vary according to such variables as age, gender, education and social class. As people get older, they are exposed to a wider variety of situations and are therefore less likely to find new situations stressful, though some older people may be resistant to change. On the other hand, younger people may perceive less danger and some may actively seek the challenge of dangerous activities. Men and women are often exposed to different types of challenge or danger during their lifetimes, acquire different skills, and demonstrate different ways of coping, and may therefore respond differently. It also appears that women are more likely than men to seek or provide social support (Matthews *et al.* 1999). People with different levels of educational attainment and job experience are likely to vary in the knowledge and skills they bring to different types of situation. Finally, those with strong social networks of family and friends are more likely to have help available than those who are socially isolated. These variables are likely to interact with each other such that those with little knowledge, skill or experience and who are socially isolated are least likely to cope successfully in new and challenging situations. But what does 'coping' actually mean?

Coping

The outcome of the appraisal process is referred to as the coping response or **coping strategy** that is used to deal with the perceived threat. Researchers have identified contrasting types of coping strategies:

- Active versus passive coping (Rosenstiel and Keefe 1983). **Active coping** refers to taking direct action to deal with the problem. **Passive coping** refers to doing nothing or relying on others to deal with it.
- Approach and avoidant coping (Miller 1992). **Approach** refers to confronting reality and dealing with problems. **Avoidance** refers to ignoring the situation or avoiding the likely consequences.
- Problem-focused and emotion-focused coping (Folkman and Lazarus 1991). **Problem-focused coping** is an active or approach strategy in which the individual actively seeks ways to mitigate or deal with a perceived threat. **Emotion-focused coping** is used to reduce the feeling of distress or fear associated with the perceived threat. This often involves avoiding having to think about or face up to it or deal with the demand or threat.

These three sets of definitions have many similarities. The best-recognized is that of Folkman and Lazarus, who drew on psychoanalytic theory to propose that emotion-focused coping is aimed primarily at managing feelings of anxiety, whereas problem-focused strategies are directed at dealing with the problem. Research findings from a variety of contexts suggest that active problem-focused strategies are related to better psychological adjustment and health outcomes than passive emotion-focused strategies.

Jo found it difficult to settle down to work again after he had left home and gone travelling. He eventually met up with Sasha, who already had a small child, Lee, and moved into her council flat. Sasha is now pregnant by Jo and they live on Sasha's social security benefits. Sasha was lonely after becoming a single parent. Lee's father had disappeared, and Sasha's mother and stepfather were not interested in helping her. Jo is a pleasant and caring young man who means well and loves having a ready-made family. But he has no idea about household management and is happy to leave all this to Sasha, who operates by crisis management. They have had a good time together buying new baby equipment and things to brighten up the flat. The debts are mounting up, but they have avoided facing up to this by transferring balances from one account to another and by taking out new loans, albeit at an exorbitant interest rate. When the debt collector arrives at the door, they pretend to be out, then have a few drinks and watch their favourite programme on their new television to cheer themselves up.

Jo and Sasha are both using emotion-focused, avoidant coping strategies. They are both trying to preserve their immediate sense of well-being by ignoring their problems and are avoiding the inevitable long-term consequences of their actions. Stress and coping is a dynamic process. The way that people cope with one problem can affect the demands on their lives in the long term. For example, the more Jo and Sasha ignore their financial problems and responsibilities, the more the problems mount up and the more difficult it becomes to find an effective way of coping.

Folkman's concept of problem-focused and emotion-focused coping has gained wide acceptance in health psychology and is widely applied in research as a convenient classification. Folkman and Lazarus (2003) identified a range of different coping strategies. We have Anglicized some of these.

- Confrontational coping: aggressive efforts to alter the situation, suggesting some degree of hostility, which could lead to identification as a 'difficult' patient.
- Distancing: cognitive efforts to detach oneself and to minimize the significance of the situation.
- Seeking social support: efforts to seek informational and emotional support and practical help.
- Escape/avoidance: wishful thinking and behavioural efforts to escape or avoid the problem.
- Problem-solving: deliberate problem-focused efforts to alter the situation, coupled with an analytic approach to solving the problem.

The selection of a particular coping strategy can be linked to the individual's sense of self-efficacy and locus of control. For example, those with an internal locus of control and sense of self-efficacy are more likely to select problem-solving coping strategies. Different coping strategies may lead to quite different outcomes if applied in similar situations. More recently, Folkman and colleagues (Park *et al.* 2001) have focused on the possibility that mental stress results from a mismatch between the type of stressor and the coping strategy used. Generally speaking, dealing with a problem by acknowledging it and trying to resolve it is better than ignoring it. But this may depend on whether or not the demand or situation is within the control of the individual or those providing support.

Review of the transactional model of stress

The Lazarus and Folkman approach to stress and coping has become very popular because it addresses cognitive and behavioural components of coping. It was adapted for nursing by Benner and Wrubel (1989), who provided a detailed analysis of the relationship between stress, coping and caring in different contexts. It is now the main theory of stress and coping in health psychology, reflecting the current emphasis on social cognition. However, below there are a number of issues that we will consider in more depth.

- The transactional model focuses on the cognitive and behavioural stress-related processes, but gives little attention to physiological processes.

- The transactional model initially gave little consideration to what is meant by the term 'threat'. More recently, Folkman and colleagues (Park *et al.* 2001) have focused on the importance of controllability.
- Some emotion-focused coping strategies, such as smoking and drinking, pose significant risks to long-term health (Chapter 8).
- Different types of social support (informational, emotional and instrumental) serve different purposes and are associated with different health outcomes.

Physiological responses to stress

In the early twentieth century, Cannon (1932) described what he termed the 'fight or flight' response. In humans, the fight or flight response occurs as an immediate reaction to a situation that is perceived as novel or potentially threatening. The response is a physiological one that involves the arousal of the autonomic nervous system and release of adrenalin. This activates the body by causing the release of glucose stored in the liver (needed for muscular activity), increasing cardiovascular activity by increasing the heart rate and blood pressure, increasing the viscosity of the blood, rerouting of blood from the digestive organs and skin to the brain and muscles, increasing the rate and depth of breathing and widening the pupils of the eyes.

Hans Selye (1956) incorporated the fight or flight response into what he termed the 'alarm reaction'. He went on to study physiological responses over time and developed a physiological model of stress called the general adaptation syndrome (GAS). The GAS has several important phases.

- The initial alarm reaction (shock) is followed by a short period of counter-shock associated with the release of adrenalin and endorphins. These increase resistance to stress by priming the body and eliminating pain in order to facilitate escape from physical threat.
- Then there is a stage of resistance in which cortisol is released into the bloodstream and resistance to stress is maintained.
- Gradually, over time, resistance to stress declines until a stage of exhaustion is reached. This is associated with the onset of stress-related illness.
- Finally, resistance to stress declines rapidly and may ultimately lead to a state of collapse, at which point the individual succumbs to disease and ultimately death.

Below, we have analysed Lazarus's stages of appraisal alongside Selye's phases of stress (see also Figure 7.1). In reality, the time span may be very variable, and the whole process influenced by such variables as genetic susceptibility.

When Mark was diagnosed as having type 2 diabetes, he experienced stress reactions that changed over time.

Primary appraisal
- Appraisal of threat (to his lifestyle and biography) and feelings of shock, accompanied by the arousal of the autonomic nervous system.
- This was followed by feelings of apprehension and anxiety, accompanied by the release of adrenalin and endorphins.

Secondary appraisal
- Mark started to think what needed to be done and what coping strategies were needed.
- Cortisol started to be released, but his immune response was strengthened.

Cycles of secondary appraisal and reappraisal
- Mark sought to establish ways of dealing with his life and the diabetes.
- He continued to feel anxious until he started to feel in control of his life with diabetes.
- Meanwhile, cortisol release was sustained and his immune response maintained.

Long-term outcomes
- Mark may find effective ways of controlling the diabetes and adapt to his changed circumstances, in which case homeostasis is restored and Mark's immune responses strengthened.
- Alternatively Mark may find no effective ways of coping with his life or his diabetes and experience a state of helplessness and hopelessness (chronic anxiety and depression), in which case his diabetes may become uncontrolled and his immune function compromised. If faced with a life-threatening disease, his body systems may be more prone to collapse and death could occur.

Stress and immune function

It has long been believed that stress leads to changes in homeostatic mechanisms that regulate heart rate and blood pressure, leading to heart disease and hypertension. More recent research has focused on the immune system. Stress has been shown to affect a number of important aspects of health, including rate of wound healing, susceptibility to infectious disease, development and progression of cancer, development and progression of autoimmune diseases, and progression of HIV infection (Kiecolt-Glaser *et al.* 2002). Kiecolt-Glaser *et al.* (2002) found that stress might compromise immune function through the following mechanisms:

- Physiological changes in the endocrine system, including the release of pituitary and adrenal hormones, as in Selye's GAS, which affect the immune system in multiple ways.
- The effects of stress-related behaviours, including tobacco, alcohol and

drug abuse, poor nutrition (e.g. comfort eating) and insufficient exercise.
- Disruption of sleep pattern.
- Anxiety and depression appear to be directly related to changes in immune response.

Findings from a variety of experiments suggest that immune function is enhanced by engagement in effortful activity (including problem-solving), perceptions of control, and social support, especially emotional and spiritual support. In contrast, exposure to uncontrollable stressors, especially prolonged exposure, compromises immune function. We address the evidence in the following sections.

Control and controllability

The concept of control has become increasingly important in research into stress and coping. Control refers to the achievement of desired outcomes. It is affected by the achievability of the goal, the controllability of the situation and the availability of resources (knowledge, skills, support) to deal with the situation. Not all situations are controllable, although most have some aspects that can be controlled.

Controllable situations

This refers to situations in which appropriate action can lead to a successful outcome. In controllable situations, the use of problem-focused coping strategies is associated with better outcomes since these are directed at resolving the problem. To ignore or avoid a demand or threat that requires direct action is not adaptive. For example, when faced with the appearance of a breast lump, ignoring it is likely to lead to a poor outcome. But sometimes the individual does not have the knowledge or skill to deal effectively with a situation that is potentially controllable. In such instances, it makes sense to seek expert help. For example, when faced with the breast lump, it makes sense to seek medical help as soon as possible in order to achieve the best outcome.

Situations such as chronic illness are often viewed as uncontrollable and can lead people to feel helpless.

When Ted went to live with Janice and Mark, they recognized that he needed to retain some independence and feel useful in spite of his limitations (he has chronic heart disease). His real love had been growing vegetables in his garden, so they bought him a large greenhouse where he could grow tomatoes, peppers, aubergines and strawberries in growing bags. This gave him something to do and made him feel a useful member of the family. This gave him back a sense of control over his life.

Uncontrollable situations

This refers to situations where outcomes are not likely to be affected by human intervention; therefore problem-focused coping strategies are of little use. A number of researchers have used certain chronic or terminal illnesses as examples of uncontrollable stressors because there is no cure and there is also a high degree of uncertainty. In such situations, it has been suggested that emotion-focused coping strategies may be more adaptive (Park *et al.* 2001). However, other researchers have found that emotion-focused coping strategies are associated with a higher level of depression in most situations.

> Sanders-Dewey (2001) examined the use of coping strategies in individuals with Parkinson's disease and their carers. They found that emotion-focused coping strategies were associated with increased psychological distress for both patients and carers. Interestingly, they found that the use of problem-focused coping by the patient was associated with a higher level of distress in the carer. This may be because attempts by their patient to manage their own condition conflict with the carer's instincts to care and protect.

Coping strategies aimed at increasing control appear more adaptive. Denial or avoidance of the reality of the situation, when used as a form of self-protection, is reported as consistently ineffective at regulating distress (Wiebe and Korbel 2003). Denial and avoidance do nothing to improve the perceived controllability of the situation. In contrast, minimizing the threat posed by the situation has been shown to reduce anxiety and maintain hope (Chapter 5). Minimizing threat is a cognitive process aimed at increasing perceived controllability. This highlights that the impact of the stressor on the individual relates to perceptions of control, rather than actual control.

Effort and controllability

Coping variables associated with overcoming challenge have been shown to be associated with positive health. Experimental evidence indicates that exposure to short-term controllable stressors involving effort enhances immune function, whereas longer-term uncontrollable stressors lead to immune depression.

> Peters *et al.* (1999) studied the effects of acute stress by presenting volunteers with a mental task in the presence of controllable or uncontrollable noise (noise increased the mental effort required to

complete the task). The researchers measured psychological, cardiovascular, endocrine and immune response. The hypothesis was that mental effort would activate the sympathetic nervous system, which would lead to an increase in immune response, specifically an increase in T and NK (natural killer) cells. The results indicated that mental effort stimulated immune response, including NK cell activity. After 15 minutes, uncontrollability led to decreased production of cytokines. The authors concluded that effort and controllability have differential effects on the immune system. Effort appears to stimulate certain aspects of immune response, while uncontrollability depresses different aspects of immune response.

The learned helplessness experiment (Chapter 4) was used to identify uncontrollability (helplessness) as a cause of gastric ulceration (Overmier and Murison 2000). Gastric ulceration is caused by the *Helicobacter pylori* infection, suggesting that a state of helplessness creates an environment in which the infection can increase. A number of researchers have studied the effects on immune function of chronic persistent (uncontrollable) stress.

Vedhara *et al.* (2002) studied the caregivers of dementia patients and found that T cell proliferation was impaired, NK cell numbers and activity were reduced, and there were elevations in herpes virus antibody titres. They then examined immune function in younger spouses of people with multiple sclerosis. In contrast to the older caregivers, they found that they were less distressed and their immune function was preserved.

One explanation is that immune function declines with age. Stress and depression are associated with greater morbidity and mortality in older adults (Kiecolt-Glaser *et al.* 2002) and it would therefore appear that older caregivers are at higher risk of illness. Another explanation for the difference between younger and older caregivers is that dementia places additional demands on caregivers and reduces emotional support.

Promoting control

Uncontrollability leads to a state of learned helplessness (Chapter 4) and is an important cause of anxiety, depression and stress-related physical illness. Uncontrollability is based on individual perceptions, and has cognitive and behavioural dimensions (Walker 2001):

- Perceived uncertainty – 'I don't know what is happening'.
- Perceived unpredictability – 'I don't know what will happen in the future'.

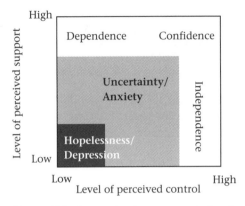

Figure 7.2   Interaction between control and support (Walker 2001).

- Perceived uncontrollability – 'I don't know what to do' or 'there is nothing that can be done'.

Uncertainty and unpredictability may be due to lack of effective knowledge or skills, but they may equally be caused by lack of adequate information. They are associated with feelings of anxiety. Knowledge deficits may be reduced or eliminated by information and education (informational social support). Sometimes, uncertainty and perceived lack of control can be due to lack of self-confidence and may respond to the provision of encouragement or emotional support. The belief that there is nothing that can be done reflects a state of hopelessness and may be associated with feelings of depression.

Because humans are social beings, there are two sources that can be used to achieve control: one's own action or help from others. Figure 7.2 demonstrates the hypothetical relationship between perceived control, perceived support and emotional state.

What happens when someone develops a persistent symptom or illness?

Janice has developed back pain. The following analysis illustrates Janice's control beliefs and emotional outcomes, given different levels of control (self-management) and/or support (medical intervention).

High control, low support. Janice successfully treats the pain without help by a combination of tablets and exercise. This strengthens her sense of self-efficacy and internal locus of control with respect to back pain.

Low control, high support. Janice cannot relieve the pain herself, so she seeks advice from an osteopath who treats it successfully. She has no personal control over the pain, but is confident that she can depend on him to relieve it in future. This reinforces external (powerful other) locus of control.

High control, high support. As well as treating the pain, the osteopath gives Janice exercises to deal with future episodes of back pain. Janice now has confidence in two alternative sources of control (internal and external powerful other).

> *Uncertain control, uncertain support.* The backache fails to respond to
> treatment and Janice searches for other sources of relief. In the
> meantime, she feels helpless and very anxious. This is typical of patients
> waiting for treatment and strengthens external (chance) locus of
> control.
> *Low control, low support.* If eventually nothing Janice or anyone else does
> seems to work, she is left feeling hopeless and depressed.

This analysis illustrates the relationship between perceived control,
perceived support and emotional outcomes.

> Ross and Mirowsky (1989: 214) conducted a large-scale American
> telephone survey. They asked people about their level of psychological
> distress, using a measure called the Center for Epidemiological Studies
> Depression Scale (CES-D) which includes items related to depression and
> anxiety. They asked some structured questions about the degree of
> control and level of support informants had in their lives. Their findings
> reflect exactly the pattern of response predicted in Figure 7.2.

Theory and research predict that perceived control and perceived support
complement each other in achieving desired outcomes and determining
emotional response. Therefore, it is not surprising that perceived support is
also an important determinant of mental and physical health.

Social support

Humans are social beings. We live in families and communities, and we
form relationships with other people in a variety of different contexts.
When faced with problems, we usually share these with others and give and
receive help. This is commonly referred to as **social support**. There is now
a large body of research that has identified social support as an important
determinant of stress-related outcomes. There are a number of different
types of social support. Some have positive effects on health, while others
can have negative effects.

- *Informational* support. This refers to the giving or receiving of information or advice that supports problem-focused coping. It been shown
  to have a positive effect on health outcomes. The advice given by a
  grandmother to a new mother about child care is one example. The
  information sheet given to a patient is another. Health care professionals
  and self-help groups are important sources of informational support with
  respect to health and illness.

- *Emotional* support. Cobb (1976) described this as information that leads individuals to feel cared for, loved and valued. Emotional support provides reassurance and encouragement. It facilitates the individual's sense of self-confidence and self-esteem and is associated with positive health.
- *Instrumental* (tangible) support. This refers to the receiving of practical help to deal with problems. It is essential at the beginning and often the end of the lifespan, and is beneficial in the short term. For example, it may involve caring for a young baby, or giving an older or disabled person assistance with housework, or driving a friend to a clinic appointment, or giving money to enable someone to receive specialist equipment. But too much practical help can lead to dependence.
- *Social affiliation/social network*. This refers to a sense of belonging. It usually involves a system of mutual obligations and reciprocal informational, emotional and instrumental social support. A social network of family and friends normally provides this. Self-help groups can also provide it. Reciprocity, giving as well as receiving help, is an important component of successful social networks.

Social support and health outcomes

Little is known about the processes through which social support affects health, but there are a number of possible positive and negative mechanisms.

- Social networks may influence whether a person comes into contact with possible disease-causing factors. For instance, a person in a stable sexual relationship is less likely to be exposed to sexually transmitted diseases than those who have many sexual partners.
- Social networks are a source of peer group pressure as well as support. For example, those with friends or relatives who engage in unhealthy lifestyles are more likely to do so themselves.
- Hobfoll (1988) suggested that people with close social networks have people around them who recognize when they are under stress or ill, and persuade them to report it to a doctor, or take a holiday, or other appropriate form of coping action.

All forms of social support are essential for children in early life. This is why Bowlby (1969) identified **attachment** relationships as being important (Chapter 5). Secure attachments appear to act as a buffer against stress (Fox and Card 1999). In addition, these early relationships may provide a template for future relationships. The lack of secure attachments leave people more susceptible to insecure relationships, stress and stress-related illnesses, including depression, throughout their lives.

Sephton *et al.* (2001) report growing evidence of links between social support, stress, emotional state, and immune and endocrine function. Social support has been shown to modulate the relationship between stress and immune function. Emotional support appears to be the most important dimension of social support (Uchino *et al.* 1996). This explains why loss of a loved one is so often associated with physical illness. Bereavement loss not only has a direct effect on the immune system, possibly because it represents a totally uncontrollable event, but also deprives people of the emotional support they would have drawn on to deal with stress (see Carman 1997).

Negative aspects of social support

Early research into social support tried to measure the perceived availability of social support in terms of quantity. People were asked about other members of their household, and whether they had neighbours and relatives living nearby. However, this proved to be of little value in understanding the relationship of social support to stress. Having people available is not enough if they are not supportive. For example, relationships that involve persistent conflict or seek to undermine the individual can have deleterious effects on physical and mental health. Other aspects of social support appear to have surprising negative effects.

Ross and Mirowsky (1989) identified from their survey that, contrary to their predictions, the more people used talking to others as a strategy for coping with stressful situations, the more depressed they tended to be. Control theory suggests that talking directed at problem-solving is likely to be beneficial. Talking aimed at grumbling or eliciting sympathy (gripe sessions) may not be beneficial.

Too much instrumental social support (practical help) has also been shown to lead to negative health outcomes because it can create passivity and dependence (Chapter 4). This suggests that control and support need to be considered together. Support aimed at solving problems and enhancing personal control is probably most beneficial.

The spiritual dimension of support

Another dimension of support is that of spiritual support. This is particularly important for those who feel helpless or hopeless, including: those with depression; those unable to find meaning or purpose in their lives; those who lack an established network of social support; and those faced with uncontrollable situations such as financial ruin, homelessness, relationship breakdown, abuse, terminal, chronic or life-threatening illness or other losses. Spirituality has been shown to reduce death anxiety (Sherman 1996). Spiritual or religious beliefs were found to be associated with increased psychological well-being in older people with chronic pain (Walker 1989; Walker et al. 1990). Spiritual support does not necessarily imply formal religious affiliation, although participation in organized religion can provide additional sources of informational, emotional and instrumental support. Spiritual support has been shown to be associated with positive health outcomes, particularly when associated with some degree of personal control.

Sephton *et al.* (2001) studied the impact of spiritual belief on immune function in women with stage IV metastatic breast carcinoma. They found that higher expression of spiritual belief was associated with higher levels of white blood cells, lymphocyte count, helper T cells, cytotoxic T cells and NK cells. Attendance at religious meetings was associated with higher lymphocyte count and immunity against infection.

There are a number of ways of explaining possible relationships between spirituality and health. In so doing, it is necessary to separate out spiritual faith from religious affiliation and religious activity. Having a spiritual faith can provide a source of emotional support that sustains confidence in times of difficulty or distress. Spirituality helps to provide a sense of meaning and coherence to life (Levin 2003; see also Chapters 2 and 5). Religious affiliations provide achievable goals. Religious activities, such as praying or reading religious texts, provide effortful coping strategies. Attendance at religious meetings provides access to a reciprocal social network that gives help in times of need.

There is some potential for psychological harm in those who expect protection from harm in exchange for religious activity or affiliation. People are often heard to say 'why me? I have done nothing wrong'. A minority of people believe that they are being punished when they become ill or disabled. This makes it difficult to predict the benefits of religion with any degree of certainty.

Emotional responses to stress

As can be seen from Figure 7.2, confidence, anxiety and depression are natural emotional responses to situations that are either controllable or uncontrollable, or are perceived as such. Most literature on stress focuses only on negative emotions, but we start with positive ones.

Confidence and pleasure

Gaining control over new or difficult situations leads to pleasure or delight and to an increase in self-confidence and self-esteem. This is particularly so when we have achieved this for ourselves. Psychologists have long recognized personal mastery as an important source of intrinsic motivation (Walker 2001). It seems also that information-processing systems may be biased to support perceptions of mastery, including exaggerated perceptions of personal control, unrealistically positive views of the self (the self-serving bias), and unrealistic optimism. The latter is associated with the belief that the present is better than the past and the future will be even better (Taylor and Brown 1988). Perhaps this helps to explain why most of us feel fairly positive most of the time.

Anxiety

Anxiety may be explained as a consequence of perceived uncertainty and unpredictability. It is often caused by extrinsic factors, such as being faced with a new or different situation where we have inadequate information. It may also be caused by intrinsic factors, such as the inability to understand or make sense of what is going on, or the lack of knowledge and skills to be able to do anything about it. These are separate from the pathological explanations given in abnormal psychology and psychiatry. Various psychological explanations for Anna's anxiety on going to university were offered in Chapter 1. You may find it interesting to re-examine these in the context of the stresses she encountered and her ability to cope with these.

Depression

Most of us feel depressed at times when nothing seems to go right, or we have experienced a severe disappointment, failure or loss. This normally subsides quickly as we regain control over our lives. Health psychologists view depressive thoughts and feelings on a continuum from absent to very severe. In contrast, when psychiatrists or clinical psychologists speak of 'depression', they usually refer to clinical depression, which is labelled using strict diagnostic criteria. Clinical depression is usually distinguished from 'ordinary' depression by its extent, severity and persistence. The following accounts are helpful in understanding how mild or severe depression might develop as a result of exposure to stressful life events and situations.

Psychodynamic accounts of depression

Psychodynamic accounts emphasize the important role of early attachment relationships and experiences of loss (Chapter 5). Insecure attachments can lead the individual to grow up with a low sense of self-esteem and poor adult relationships. There is support in the literature for the notion that adults who have secure attachment relationships are less vulnerable to depression following adverse life events. This is equally true for those with intellectual disabilities and may also account for some behavioural problems.

Janssen *et al.* (2002) reviewed studies of stress, coping and attachment in people with intellectual disability (ID). They found evidence that intellectually disabled people were more vulnerable to stress and use less effective coping strategies. Studies of attachment indicate that people with ID are at risk of developing insecure or disorganized attachment. This may put them at risk of developing challenging behaviours, particularly when faced with stressful situations or life change.

Cognitive theories of depression

Beck (1976) proposed that the beliefs of people who are depressed are distorted in a negative direction. He suggested that experiences of loss or failure lead people to reflect inwardly on what they have done wrong and blame themselves. His cognitive approach to therapy involves cognitive restructuring, aimed at encouraging positive thinking. However, Taylor and Brown (1988) demonstrated that the negative beliefs of people who are depressed are actually realistic. It is people who are not depressed who hold illusions of control and are unrealistically optimistic. Nevertheless, positive thinking remains an important component of cognitive behavioural therapy. Beck is probably best known for his Beck Depression Inventory (Beck *et al.* 1997) which is probably the most widely used measure of depression used in research.

Behaviourist accounts of depression

Learned helplessness
This account of depression was described in Chapter 4. According to Seligman (1975), depression reflects a sense of helplessness or hopelessness. It is a response to perceived uncontrollability, in which the individual learns that their actions have no effect on outcomes. The treatment of depression, based on this account, is to demonstrate to the individual that their actions can influence outcomes. Therapy starts with small achievable actions with guaranteed positive outcomes. Further graded tasks, starting with easy ones and building up to more complex ones, are then agreed based on the principle that success breeds success.

Behavioural theories of depression
Lewinsohn (1974) noted that those who are depressed have little positive social reinforcement in their lives. Reasons for this include social isolation, bereavement and poverty. Based on this model, it was proposed that treatment for depression needed to focus on increasing positive reinforcement. Since most people gain positive reinforcement in social situations, therapy included teaching social skills and finding new social networks.

Who gets anxious and depressed?

The 'Whitehall study' of all grades of British civil servants produced the following findings (Griffin *et al.* 2002):

- A greater proportion of women than men were classed as depressed or anxious.
- Younger women and men were more likely to be depressed than working people who were older.
- Women with low control at home were more than twice at risk of depression than women with high control, even after controlling for marital status, number of children, and caregiving status.
- Low home control increased men's risk of depression.

- Men who were caregivers consistently had a significantly higher risk for depression and anxiety.

Mirowsky and Ross (2003) explained gender differences in psychological distress (anxiety and depression) by the degree of control women have over their lives in comparison to men, including the division of responsibility and labour within the home. Their survey showed that marriage seems particularly important for the mental health of men, probably because of the quality of the supportive relationship many marriages provide.

Individual differences in responses to stress

It has always been recognized that people vary in their responses to stress. Therefore, psychologists have been interested in identifying stable differences in personality or coping style that could account for differences in susceptibility to stress-related illness. A number of possibilities have been studied.

Optimism versus pessimism

It is clear that people vary in the ways they view similar situations. Some people regard life events as challenges; others see them as threats. Some view their cup as half full and others as half empty. A number of studies suggest that optimists have better psychological adjustment and immune responses to stressful life events than pessimists.

Brissette *et al.* (2002) suggested that optimists use more effective coping strategies and have more supportive social networks, and that this is why optimists are usually found to be less prone to stress (though it is difficult to distinguish between cause and effect). Cohen *et al.* (1999) compared the immune responses of optimists and pessimists to acute and chronic stressors. They found that optimists had better immune function following acute stress, whereas pessimists showed no effect. But in situations of persistent high stress, optimists showed more immune depression than pessimists.

A possible explanation is that optimists are optimistic because they tend to deal successfully with situations. They are therefore more likely to view demands as challenges and put more effort into achieving mastery. But in the face of longer-term uncontrollable stressors, optimists experience a greater sense of helplessness and failure, whereas pessimists get what they expected. Although optimism and pessimism are somewhat stable over time, they reflect expectations that can change in the light of experience.

Type A and Type C personalities

In the 1970s, there appeared to emerge evidence for a Type A behaviour pattern or 'coronary prone personality' that consisted of sense of time urgency, competitiveness and aggressiveness (Friedman and Rosenman, 1974). In the 1980s, a Type C behaviour pattern (passivity, compliance and suppression of anger) was identified as being associated with cancer proneness or poor survival rates (Temoshok, 1987). Subsequent research has failed to find support for these concepts. More recent evidence suggests that hostility and anger lead to increased health risk in men, but not women. It has been suggested that anger is associated with the failure to gain control, and may also reflect a lower ability to benefit from social support (Kivimäki *et al.* 2003).

Hardy personality

Kobasa (1979) introduced the concept of the 'hardy' personality which consisted of a set of characteristics, the three Cs, associated with protection from stress-related illness:

• Commitment – active involvement in life activities.
• Control – a belief in the ability to influence life events.
• Challenge – a belief that change is normal and growth-enhancing.

Several studies have confirmed that hardiness is associated with increased immune function (Dolbier *et al.* 2001). Nicholas (1993) found that those scoring high on hardy characteristics were more likely to engage in good self-care behaviours. They are therefore less susceptible to illness caused by smoking, alcohol, poor diet or lack of exercise. Hardy characteristics appear to reflect a combination of internal locus of control and optimism.

The 'Big Five'

Research into the relationship between the 'Big Five' personality factors and stress has not proved particularly useful. These issues were discussed in Chapter 2.

Locus of control

Associations between internal and external locus of control dimensions (Chapter 4) and health outcomes tend to be consistent, though fairly weak:

• Internal locus of control is associated with the use of active, problem-focused coping. Those with internal locus of control are more likely to take direct action to protect health and engage in self-management of chronic disease. For example, Härkäpää *et al.* (1991) found that patients with low back pain who had internal control beliefs learned their exercises better and did their exercises more frequently.

- External (powerful others) locus of control may also be associated with problem-focused coping if it leads people to seek appropriate informational support. Powerful others locus of control is not adaptive if it leads to dependence on others.
- External (chance) locus of control is the opposite of internal locus of control. Those who believe that what happens to them is a matter of luck, fate or chance are likely to be fatalistic, less likely to engage in health-protective behaviours and more likely to engage in avoidant coping strategies. Research consistently shows that chance locus of control is associated with inaction and poor health outcomes.

Sense of coherence

Antonovsky (1985) proposed 'sense of coherence' as a key predictor of long-term mental and physical health. This means seeing the world as rational, predictable, controllable and meaningful. Items taken from a scale constructed to measure sense of coherence include such issues as the belief that daily activities give pleasure and that life in future will be full of meaning and purpose (Bowling 1997). Sense of coherence has been shown to be associated with successful ageing and with a range of positive health consequences, including immune function and pain tolerance. Stressful life events, illnesses or losses disrupt an individual's biographical coherence (Chapters 2 and 5).

Individual differences and stress-related illness

Not all people who are stressed develop stress-related disease. It has long been recognized that many diseases associated with stress, including heart disease, are influenced by family history. Some of this influence may be accounted for by family patterns of coping behaviour. However, genetic susceptibility is likely to be an important factor (Marsland *et al.* 2002).

Marsland *et al.* (2002) examined immune response to simulated daily hassles, using mental arithmetic and public speaking, and found a wide range of individual responses. Those who demonstrated a high level of sympathetic response to the tasks showed stress-induced increases in cytotoxic T cell activity. Their findings confirm that some people are more prone to stress and stress-related illness than others for reasons associated with their physiological responses.

Review of personality and stress

Overall, it is well recognized that individual differences in physical and emotional responses to stress exist. However, the notion of the stress-prone personality has not proved helpful, as associations with health outcomes tend to be weak. Patterns of belief, expectations and behaviours associated with stress protection include those identified as part of Kobasa's hardy personality. These are: perceived control, commitment or conscientiousness, challenge or optimism. Sense of coherence is related to sense of controllability and is associated with resistance to stress and positive health outcomes. Chance locus of control is associated with poor health outcomes. Neuroticism is a measure of emotional stability and is highly correlated with adverse psychological outcomes. Expressed hostility and anger are associated with increased vulnerability to stress-related illness in men, in whom it reflects lack of appropriate coping strategies and leads to poor social support. Overall, many of these factors appear to relate to the capacity of the individual to gain or maintain personal control over situations in which they find themselves.

Stress in different contexts

Illness and hospitalization

When people are ill, their immune systems are often compromised or under strain. It is therefore particularly important to help people find ways of reducing uncertainty and unpredictability, enhance personal control, and provide appropriate informational, emotional and instrumental support. Information-giving and patient education are essential to reducing uncertainty and unpredictability and increasing controllability in health care settings. Even when problems seem overwhelming, health care professionals can help patients to identify aspects of their situation that they can control. When someone has developed a chronic illness or disability, they need time to mourn their loss and identify short-term achievable goals.

Janice's friend, Mike, attended the out-patient department complaining of pain. He had a congenital deformity and had recently had both hips replaced. Although the operations were successful, he complained of pain 'everywhere' and appeared depressed. Mike explained he had always been very fit. But after his hip operations, he watched old ladies getting up and going home while he could hardly move. This made him feel helpless. The pain consultant suggested that Mike needed to focus on exercises to regain cardiovascular fitness, since this would also increase the circulation of endorphins and help to reduce his pain. At his next appointment, Mike reported that the pain was now controllable and he was feeling optimistic. At the end of six months, his business was flourishing and his partner was expecting their baby. He had focused on the short-term goal of regaining fitness.

Patient education and self-management programmes aimed at increasing self-efficacy and personal control are essential to stress management of chronic illness (Chapter 8).

Lund and Tamm (2001) conducted a qualitative study in Sweden into the process of adjustment in elderly people who had been ill and undergone rehabilitation, but remained disabled. They found that initial care focused on physical rehabilitation and involved interaction with health care professionals. Following this, participants reported a period in which they struggled to come to terms with what had happened and find new meaning in their lives. As time progressed, they had to negotiate changes in interpersonal relationships and deal with stigmatizing attitudes in their daily lives. Lund and Tamm commented that although professionals in Sweden claimed rehabilitation took a holistic approach, participants received little help or support in dealing with these psychosocial aspects of change.

Life events

Holmes and Rahe (1967) developed a measure of life events called the Social Readjustment Rating Scale (SRRS; Homes and Rahe, 1967). It consisted of 43 common positive and negative life-changing events, ranked in order of importance. Marriage was given an arbitrary score of 50. Loss of a spouse was presumed to be most stressful and was given a score of 100. The SRRS proved a popular tool because it was simple and easy to use. But it is now seriously out of date and fails to take account of the many cultural changes that affect perceptions of stress.

Some evidence supported a link between life events and subsequent illness, but generally the correlation (a statistical measure of association) was low and the results disappointing. An important reason may be that the SRRS fails to distinguish between events that are controllable and those that are uncontrollable. In addition, the notion of a direct association between life events and stress-related illness overlooks the fact that many stress-related illnesses are caused by maladaptive coping responses, such as smoking, drinking excess alcohol, or comfort eating.

Events involving loss, such as death, trauma or job loss, often involve loss of control over one's life and loss of support. It is therefore helpful to assess if patients have experienced these, find out how they are coping with them and what support, including listening, might be helpful.

Daily hassles

People who have had relatively little exposure to major life events may nevertheless be susceptible to the development of stress-related illness. 'Daily hassles' refers to the accumulation of the minor annoying things like missing the bus, being late for work or spilling the coffee. A considerable volume of research suggests that daily hassles are indeed associated with depression.

People who are disadvantaged through poverty or have a chronic illness experience a much greater number of what Hewison (1997) observed to be cumulative hassles and recurrent crises. These include negotiating with benefits agencies and hospital systems, while attempting to deal with financial and various other losses and relationship problems (Walker *et al.* 1999). A good way of finding out the types of hassles that patients experience is to listen to their accounts of health care, observe reactions during episodes of care or read qualitative research reports of patient experiences of care. Many hassles can easily be reduced and stress diminished, leading to improvements in patient satisfaction and health.

Traumatic events and post-traumatic stress disorder

It has long been recognized that a single catastrophic event can lead to a mental health condition called post-traumatic stress disorder (PTSD). According to the DSM-IV, the diagnostic manual for mental health (American Psychiatric Association 2000), PTSD may occur if the person has been exposed to the trauma of experiencing, witnessing, or being confronted with actual or threatened death or serious injury, or a threat to the physical integrity of self or others and responded with intense fear, helplessness, or horror. PTSD has been recorded in response to a variety of events including assault, accident, disaster and medical treatment. Symptoms of PTSD include:

- Recurrent and intrusive distressing recollections of the event, including images, thoughts, and/or perceptions. In young children, repetitive play may occur in which these or other aspects of the trauma are expressed.
- Recurrent distressing dreams of the event. In young children, there may be frightening dreams without recognizable content.
- A sense of reliving the experience, illusions, hallucinations, and/or flashbacks, including those that occur on awakening or when intoxicated. In young children, trauma-specific re-enactment may occur.
- Intense psychological distress and/or physiological reactivity on exposure to internal or external cues that symbolize or resemble an aspect of the traumatic event.

Typically, the individual persistently tries to avoid thoughts, conversations or recall of memories associated with the trauma and experiences a sense of emotional numbness or detachment. Other symptoms include at least two of the following:

- difficulty falling or staying asleep;
- irritability or outbursts of anger;
- difficulty concentrating;
- hypervigilance;
- exaggerated startle response.

Symptoms may occur immediately following the trauma, or may be delayed. Most recover within a few weeks or months without treatment, particularly if there is good family support. Ehlers and Clark (2000) suggested that memories of the traumatic event are poorly encoded in long-term memory because things happened so quickly. As a result, victims are unable to control their responses or make sense or meaning out of what happened. They are therefore unable to integrate the event or their response to it into biographical memory.

Treatment of PTSD

It was originally believed that immediate counselling was important in the prevention of PTSD. However, a meta-analysis of all studies of psychological debriefing indicated that debriefing *increased* the risk of PTSD nearly three-fold (Rose *et al.* 2004). Therefore the current advice is that compulsory debriefing after trauma should stop. That is not to say that people should be discouraged from talking about the event to family, friends or confidants if they wish to do so.

Health care professionals need to warn people who have experienced a traumatic incident that it is possible they may at some time in the future experience flashbacks associated with feelings of panic. Patients can be reassured that most of the symptoms disappear within three months, but if they do not then their doctor should refer them for treatment to a clinical psychologist who specializes in PTSD. Treatment involves cognitive behavioural therapy, of which systematic desensitization (Chapter 4) is likely to be a component. This requires the patient to consciously hold images of the trauma in their mind until sympathetic arousal has subsided and they feel calm. When done repeatedly, the conditioned fear response associated with traumatic memories is eliminated. It is helpful if people talk about the event following treatment to prevent recurrence.

Organizational stress

Much of our life is spent at work, and the working environment has proved an interesting source of research into stress and stress-related illness. It used to be thought that stress was a result of work pressure and was therefore associated with the high-flying executive (such as a senior hospital manager). But more recent research has demonstrated that this is not the case. The most systematic study of work-related stress is the 'Whitehall study', an intensive study of British civil servants.

Theories of organizational stress tested as part of the study include the 'demand–control–support' and 'effort–reward imbalance' models. Findings indicate that effort–reward imbalance (people do not get what they think they deserve) and low job control are related to the incidence of coronary heart disease (Marmot 1999). Family life, social support and leisure activities are important buffers against the effects of work-related stress. Stansfield (1999) observed that since social support plays an important role in preventing physical and psychological morbidity, interventions to improve social cohesion at work are important.

A few years ago, Mark was working from home as a regional sales representative for a firm selling office supplies. But he had become increasingly anxious and depressed and was eventually signed off sick with 'depression'. He received help from a counsellor. A brief initial analysis revealed that his stress was probably job-related. His pay depended on sales and he invested a high level of effort for relatively little return. He felt he had little job control and was swamped with paperwork. He had no colleague or supervisor support since the office base was 50 miles away. High effort and low reward, plus high demand, low job control and low job support equals high stress. Mark resigned from the job and his depression lifted immediately. He obtained a less demanding and more autonomous job as a groundsman, working with a team of others, which he loved.

Health care services expose employees at all levels to high levels of demand, but with varying degrees of job control and support. Stress is increased when staff have personal, financial or health problems, or lack adequate emotional support outside work. The problem of **burnout** has long been recognized among the caring professions. This is where stress leads to low job satisfaction, poor performance and a lack of ability to empathize with patients as staff are no longer able to cope with the emotional demands of caring. Support groups for staff are an increasingly popular method of supporting professional carers. These need careful facilitation to provide emotional and problem-solving support and avoid negativity.

The management of stress

The first aim of stress management should be to assess the number, nature and controllability of the stressors faced by the individual, and identify if they are using effective ways of coping. Help to deal with the stressor might, for example, involve job relocation or retraining, or marital or financial guidance, which would require referral to appropriate agencies. Stress management courses emphasize the development of coping skills, such as prioritizing, time management and organizational or assertiveness skills. If stress-related problems are caused by relationship problems or the failure to come to terms with past events, counselling may be helpful. A counsellor can also help the individual to review their goals and help them to focus on achievable aims. For those with more severe anxiety problems, such as PTSD, cognitive behavioural therapy uses psychological principles to improve the ability of the individual to confront and deal successfully with life stresses (Chapter 4). In the next chapter we review the principles of self-management that also aim to reduce stress for people with chronic illnesses or disabilities.

Summary of key points

- Stress involves an interaction between a stressor, the perceived ability of the individual to achieve a desired outcome, and the individual's coping response.
- Effective coping strategies are those that enhance sense of control and immune function. These include problem-focused, active and effortful coping when used in controllable situations.
- Supports that protect against stress include informational support (advice, information and guidance), emotional support (loving, caring) and spiritual support.
- Anxiety, depression and anger are natural emotional responses to stress.
- Physiological and immune responses to stress are closely associated with its positive and negative emotional consequences.
- Traumatic and other major life events (particularly those involving loss), daily hassles (particularly when associated with poverty and deprivation), illness and hospitalization, and organization in the workplace are all important sources of stress and stress-related illness.

Further reading

Cameron, L.D. and Leventhal, H. (eds) (2003) *The Self-Regulation of Health and Illness Behaviour*. London: Routledge.

Marmot, M. and Wilkinson, R.G. (eds) (1999) *Social Determinants of Health*: Oxford: Oxford University Press.

Mirowsky, J. and Ross, C.E. (2003) *Social Causes of Psychological Distress*, 2nd edition. New York: Aldine de Gruyter.

Walker J. (2001) *Control and the Psychology of Health*. Buckingham: Open University Press, Chapter 8.

PSYCHOLOGY APPLIED TO HEALTH AND WELL-BEING

- What do we mean by the terms 'health', 'illness' and 'quality of life', and how can they be measured?
- What is meant by social cognition, and why are social cognitive theories important when assessing and planning health-promoting interventions?
- What are the main reasons why people fail to take health advice, and how can we improve this?
- Why is it difficult to predict with any certainty whether or not people will change their behaviour, even when they want to?
- Why is it important to identify key individual goals when planning self-management strategies?
- What do lay teachers have to contribute to self-management programmes?
- What quick and simple outcome measures are useful to evaluate clinical interventions?

Introduction

This chapter focuses on the application of psychology to the promotion of positive health and well-being, and the prevention and management of ill health. The concepts of 'health' and 'illness' reflect subjective beliefs and experience. Therefore, in clinical practice, these need to be understood from the perspective of each individual patient. Nevertheless, there are commonalities of belief and experience that have been used to build theories that can help to guide assessment and interventions. The theories used to explain health-related beliefs and predict health-related behaviours are termed **social cognitive theories**. Social cognition combines theoretical positions from cognitive science, social learning and social psychology to identify factors likely to influence health-related behaviours and behaviour change. These enable health care professionals to assess the likelihood that an individual will engage in or change health-related behaviours and identify barriers to health action. They also guide the development of interventions likely to promote health and well-being.

Social cognition models are explored here in the context of primary, secondary and tertiary prevention, and are related to the behaviours of patients and health care professionals. We also examine principles of self-management, in contrast to those of compliance or adherence, for those who have enduring health problems. Ways of measuring and evaluating health outcomes in practice are considered. **Health-related behaviours** are those that affect health and illness, but are usually engaged in for reasons other than their health effects.

Defining health, illness and disease

The most widely cited definition of 'health' was provided by the World Health Organization (WHO) in 1948. It has since officially remained unchanged, although it is now emphasized that health is a dynamic and not a static state: 'Health is a state of complete physical, mental and social well-being, not merely the absence of disease or infirmity' (WHO 2004a).

It is helpful to distinguish between illness and disease. Eisenberg (1977) suggested that patients experience illness, while doctors diagnose and treat disease. Similarly, Blaxter (1990) defined 'disease' as a biological or clinically identified abnormality, and 'illness' as the subjective experience of symptoms. Therefore, she argued, it is possible to have an illness without a disease, and a disease without being ill.

Mark has hypertension, which is a disease associated with high blood pressure. It is an important cause of heart disease, stroke and kidney failure and places Mark at high risk of further health problems. But hypertension usually remains symptom-free until the late stages and is therefore an example of disease without illness. This makes it difficult for Mark to perceive it as a problem.

It is important to note that definitions of illness and disease used here are based on the assumptions of western biomedical science. Alternative explanations and effective approaches to the treatment of illness are to be found outside medicine, including eastern traditions and complementary therapies. These are particularly relevant in cases of illness that are not associated with a disease that is clearly identifiable, and treatable or preventable. For example, the cause of chronic back pain is extremely difficult to diagnose, but many people find that their back pain responds to osteopathy, acupuncture, meditation or Pilates, even though the evidence base for some of these treatments is somewhat limited (Bandolier 2004). Alternative and complementary therapies provide a powerful vehicle for the benefits of the therapeutic relationship, as well as any direct therapeutic effects.

Closely associated with health is the concept of 'quality of life'. For any individual at a particular time, quality of life may lie somewhere on a continuum between a complete state of well-being and a state of absolute wretchedness. While the opposite of 'health' is usually considered to be 'illness', the opposite of 'well-being' may or may not include illness, disease or infirmity. Grief may be regarded as such an example (Chapter 5). Quality of life is a multifactorial concept that includes physical, mental, functional, social and spiritual well-being. In fact, it embraces health in its broadest definition.

It is difficult to define someone as either healthy or ill because these are relative concepts. Many older people who experience infirmities common in later life nevertheless regard themselves as healthy. Medical diagnoses change as medical technologies improve. Mental health provides a good example of how medical explanations and treatments change over time, even in the absence of new technologies. Diagnosis of mental illness is based on symptom classification, which is subject to cultural changes in attitude as well as knowledge. For example, homosexuality used to be classified as a mental illness, while bulimia nervosa was not recognized as a mental health disorder until the 1970s. Mental health classifications sometimes respond to political demands. Drapetomania (the tendency of slaves to run away from their masters) in nineteenth-century America and political dissidence in the twentieth-century USSR are examples. The more recent classification of 'personality disorder' in the UK might be seen by some as a political response to the management of asocial behaviour. A useful account of some of these issues is provided by the WHO (2001).

Cross-cultural and lay explanations of physical and mental health vary widely, and it is essential to take account of these understandings when working with people from different cultural traditions. An exploration of these issues is to be found within the sociology of health and illness, and provides important contextual information for understanding the psychology of health and illness. For the purposes of this chapter, we focus on the psychology of health and illness in the context of western medicine and health care systems.

Promoting health and preventing ill health

When considering how to apply psychology to health, it is important to distinguish between three distinct types of activity:

- the avoidance of disease, known as primary prevention;
- early detection and treatment to arrest a disease process already initiated, known as secondary prevention;
- rehabilitation and symptom management to restore the individual to their previous level of function or maximize their remaining capacities, known as tertiary prevention (see Leavell and Clark 1965; WHO 2001).

In this chapter, we focus on each aspect of prevention, drawing mainly on social cognitive theories.

Social cognition

Social cognition is concerned with how individuals make sense of social situations (Conner and Norman 1995). Humans are social beings and have relationships of interdependence with others at many different levels at home, at work, at leisure, and in society. Social cognitive theories focus on the thoughts or beliefs that lead to health-related behaviours or behaviour change in particular social contexts. Cognitive theories are based on the assumption that there is a causal chain between beliefs, attitudes and behaviour, as illustrated in Figure 8.1. (This assumption is rejected by radical behaviourists who argue in favour of a direct relationship between external stimuli and behaviour; see Chapter 4.) The 'external stimuli' in the context of Figure 8.1 refer to such things as health messages, media images, health advice, illness symptoms, family and peer influence, all of which need to be understood within the social and cultural context of the individual or group of individuals concerned.

Social cognition and prevention

In this section, we focus particularly on behaviours which, if changed, would lead to a significant reduction in mortality and morbidity within the population (Department of Health (DoH) 1999). It is important to set this in the context of key contemporary public health issues, in order to identify behaviours associated with health risk (see Figure 8.2).

The main causes of mortality and morbidity in western populations include heart disease, stroke and cancer (DoH 1999). Important risk behaviours associated with these diseases include smoking, eating a diet high in saturated fats and low in fruit and vegetables, and taking too little exercise. Behaviours associated with risk reduction (primary prevention) are therefore cessation of smoking, change of diet and increase in exercise. Secondary prevention focuses on attendance for cancer screening (e.g. cervical screening and mammography) as well as attending for screening for diabetes, high blood pressure and hyperlidipaemia. These behaviours are priorities for health professionals.

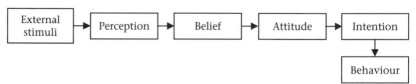

Figure 8.1 Chain of causal assumptions associated with cognitive theories.

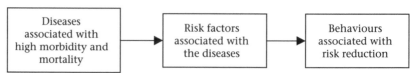

Figure 8.2 Identifying 'risky' health-related behaviours.

Health psychologists use social cognitive theories and models in an attempt to predict the likelihood of that people will comply with health advice. The best-known and most widely used by health care professionals is the health belief model.

The health belief model (HBM)

The health belief model (HBM) is what is termed in psychology an 'expectancy-value' model. This means that it assumes that action is based on a cognitive evaluation of the outcome of a particular behaviour or behaviour change. The HBM was originally developed by Hochbaum in the 1950s, at a time when tuberculosis was an important health problem, in order to understand why so many people failed to attend for chest X-ray screening (Rosenstock 1974a). The HBM was reported by Rosenstock (1974b), reviewed by Becker and Maiman (1975), modified by Janz and Becker (1984) and extended by Rosenstock *et al.* (1988). It has proved a popular and durable model within health education. Its components are given in Figure 8.3.

Applying the HBM to change of diet, it is proposed that we are more likely to make a change if:

- we feel that failure to change exposes us to the risk of getting a disease that could have serious consequences for us.
- the benefits of making the change outweigh the barriers to change. The barriers include psychological barriers, such as perceived lack of ability to achieve the change (perceived self-efficacy).
- we value our health sufficiently to be motivated to make the effort to change (health value).
- we are prompted to change by external cues, such as health messages, advice, information, or the development of symptoms (cues to action).

The model predicts that the more vulnerable we feel ourselves to be to a disease that would have severe consequences, the more likely we are to take

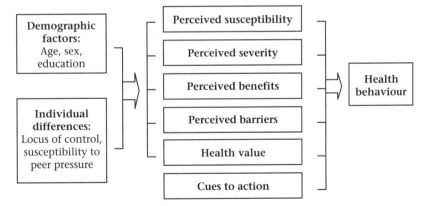

Figure 8.3 The health belief model (adapted from Rosenstock 1974b; Rosenstock *et al.* 1988).

the action necessary to avoid the disease or its consequences. These beliefs are influenced by demographic factors and individual differences, as well as knowledge and experience. But even if we perceived ourselves to be vulnerable, we still need to see that the benefits of behaviour change will outweigh the difficulties involved in making the change.

> Before Jo moved in with Sasha, Anna was very concerned about his diet because he lived on pizza and other convenience foods, and refused to eat fresh fruit or vegetables. Anna used the health belief model to assess the likelihood that he would change his diet. Jo did not believe that his diet placed him at risk, could see no benefits to changing, and identified a range of barriers including his food preferences, time to buy and prepare healthy foods, and peer group pressure to eat pizza. He was aware of health messages (cues) in the media, but did not feel that they were relevant to him. He believed that heart disease was a disease of older people and took his own health for granted. Anna concluded that it was unlikely he would change to a healthy diet in his present situation.

Review of the health belief model

The HBM was developed from interviews about screening attendance, and this explains the disease focus of the model. Screening attendance is part of secondary prevention (early detection of disease) and involves a single action directed towards disease prevention. It is therefore legitimate to claim a causal link between health beliefs and health behaviour. However, the HBM has since been applied as part of primary prevention to a range of lifestyle activities such as smoking, eating, drinking, exercise and sexual activity. These behaviours are clearly related to health from a public health perspective, but not necessarily in the minds of people at the time they engage in them (Galvin 1992). People smoke, eat, drink and engage in sexual activity because they give pleasure or have other reinforcing effects (Chapter 4). Therefore, the HBM may be less relevant in explaining these health-related behaviours and behaviour change.

The most important reasons for failure to change lifestyle behaviours have been identified as perceived vulnerability and barriers to implementation (Sheeran and Abraham 1995). Those who do not believe themselves to be vulnerable are unlikely to take any notice of health promotion campaigns. But barriers prevent change, even when motivation is high and intentions to change strong. Barriers refer to all factors likely to reduce, limit or inhibit a health-promoting response. Many of these involve social pressures that are unforeseen at the time of making a commitment to change. Therefore, if the HBM is to be a useful aid to patient assessment, it is essential to encourage the individual to think through all possible environmental, social and psychological barriers likely to interfere with their ability to make specific changes (see Chapter 4).

The theory of planned behaviour (TPB)

Ajzen and Fishbein (1980) designed the theory of reasoned action (TRA) to explain any behaviour, including buying a car, choosing a shirt or smoking a particular brand of cigarette. Later, Ajzen (1988, 1991) added the additional variable 'perceived behavioural control' to increase the power of the TRA to predict behaviour, and changed the name to the theory of planned behaviour (TPB). The TPB (Figure 8.4) is currently the most popular and most widely used social cognition model in health psychology.

The TPB is based on the assumption that health-related behaviours are under conscious or voluntary control. According to the theory, the intention to behave in a certain way, or to change a behaviour, is determined by three factors:

- Attitude towards the behaviour. This reflects a value judgement about whether or not the individual thinks the behaviour is a good thing. It is based on an evaluation about the desirability of the outcome of the proposed action.
- The 'subjective norm'. This refers to the individual's beliefs about what others who are important to them think they should do, together with their motivation to comply with these wishes.
- Perceived behavioural control. This refers to an assessment of the degree of control individuals perceive themselves to have over the particular action. It is based on an appraisal of the individual about whether or not they have the necessary skills, abilities and resources to achieve the behaviour. It is similar to Bandura's concept of self-efficacy (Chapter 4),

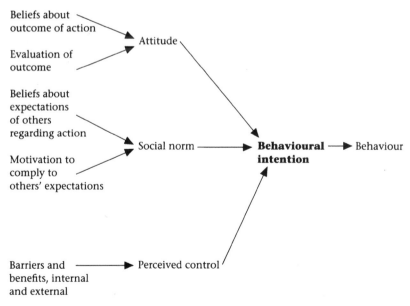

Figure 8.4 The theory of planned behaviour (adapted from Ajzen 1991).

but also takes account of available resources, such as money, social support and opportunity.

Janice has had an invitation to attend for a mammogram and is deciding whether or not to attend.

- *Attitude*. Janice believes that attending for screening will have positive benefits. If it proves negative, it will reassure her. If it proves positive, it will enable her to receive early treatment for breast cancer and this will improve the outcome for her.
- *Subjective or social norm*. Janice believes that her family would wish her to attend for screening. Her friends all attend and expect her to do the same.
- *Perceived behavioural control*. It is quite easy for Janice to attend for screening as the unit comes to her workplace. She will need to change the appointment to fit in with her shift at work, but the contact details make it easy for her to do this. She knows about the procedure and is not frightened about what will happen.

In this situation, the model predicts that Janice intends to attend for mammogram and is likely to carry out her intention unless there is an unforeseen obstacle, such as illness or the car breaking down. However, the analysis is more difficult when applied to a lifestyle behaviour, such as smoking, drinking, eating or exercise, where external influences are greater and change more difficult to put into action.

Mark was advised by the cardiologist to walk for at least 20 minutes per day, but has so far failed to do this. He believes that exercise would do him good (positive attitude). Janice and Anna want him to do it (subjective norm). He knows that he could easily do it if he wanted to (perceived behavioural control) because he has the ability and the resources (clothes, shoes, pathways) to do it. Therefore he really intends to it. But somehow, he keeps putting it off until tomorrow when the weather is better, or he has more time.

The TPB does not appear sufficiently robust to detect why Mark has not so far implemented his intention. Research with the TPB indicates that the model is reasonable good at predicting intentions (Ajzen, 1991) but less good at predicting actual behaviour. A recent meta-analysis of research findings suggests that the TPB accounts for about 39% of the variance for intention and 27% of the variance for behaviour (Armitage and Conner 2001). These percentages are estimates of the explanatory power of the model. The most important variable is perceived behavioural control, which in many instances is shown to have a direct influence on behaviour as well as intention. But the longer the gap between expressing intentions and taking action, the less likely it is that the action will take place. Therefore an immediate demonstration of commitment is desirable. Once again, unforeseen barriers are probably important in preventing people from carrying out their good intentions.

Critique of the HBM and TPB

These two social cognition models provided the basis for much of health psychology practice and research in relation to primary and secondary prevention in the 1990s. The TPB has proved to be the most popular model because of its versatility in explaining a wide range of behaviours. But even this has proved to be at best modest in predicting actual behaviour. There are a number of possible reasons for this.

Unlike behaviourist learning theory, social cognition models assume that health-related behaviours are based upon rational processes of reasoning and deliberation. This is reasonable when applied to the decision to engage in a one-off action like attending for screening. But most lifestyle behaviours that influence long-term health outcomes, such as eating, drinking and smoking, are habits. Habits are, by definition, things that we do routinely, without thinking. Using the language of behaviourism, these behaviours are under stimulus control (Chapter 4). They are therefore hard to change even when we want to do so.

Hunt and Martin (1988) provided a useful analysis of lifestyle behaviours. They suggested that daily life needs some kind of interruption to bring an existing habit or lifestyle into conscious focus, so that it can be changed. An example might be meeting a new partner who does not smoke, or moving to a new area with a new set of friends. They also suggest that new behaviours, such as taking up exercise, are unlikely to be maintained until they have become habits and take place without having to think too hard about them.

Social cognition models do not distinguish between different types of behaviour change. For example, smoking, drinking and substance use are behaviours that need to stop. Therefore, some other activity needs to be introduced to compensate for the time spent engaged in these activities (Chapter 4). Exercise involves the introduction of a new behaviour that needs to displace some other activity or routine. Dietary change involves substitution. This is not difficult provided the displaced activity is not seen as more desirable than the new activity. For example, going out to take exercise may be seen as less desirable by Mark than relaxing in front of the television. Therefore, each behaviour needs careful analysis in relation to the change process.

Many health-related behaviours are actually coping strategies used for dealing with stress. Smoking, comfort eating and drinking alcohol are good examples. Therefore, it will be difficult to change if the individual is under stress, unless equally good alternative coping strategies are available. People often fail to take account of this at the time they express an intention to change. Stress may therefore be an important barrier to behaviour change, but is often omitted from consideration in the literature.

An important criticism of social cognition models is their lack of emphasis on the immediate and unforeseen social consequences of the behaviour.

> Coleman and Ingham (1999) interviewed young people about their use of contraception. They found that first sexual experiences were usually unplanned and protection therefore not used. The association of a condom with disease prevention could actually inhibit use, since using a condom or asking a partner to use a condom might imply lack of trust. Coleman and Ingham discussed this in relation to the need for enhanced communication skills.

Ingham (1993) criticized the use of cognitive models because these fail to take account of the social situations in which the behaviours occur. For example, he suggested in relation to sexual behaviour that when the lights are low, the alcohol flowing, and passions rising, good intentions are inclined to be forgotten.

Some authors have recommended combining models to strengthen the ability to predict health behaviours (e.g. Maddux 1993). This allows for the identification of psychological and social barriers likely to reduce self-efficacy at the point of action. Another recommended approach is to assess readiness to adopt a behaviour change.

Stages of change

Prochaska and DiClemente (1983) recognized that an important determinant of health-related behaviour change, particularly in relation to smoking cessation, was the readiness of the individual to change. They produced the stages of change model (also called the 'transtheoretical model') that is useful when planning the most appropriate approach to intervention. The stages of change they identified were as follows:

- *Pre-contemplation.* At this stage, the individual is not considering change and may not even recognize the need for change.
- *Contemplation.* The individual has recognized a need to change and is starting to think about possible ways of achieving this.
- *Action planning.* The individual is planning how to make the change.
- *Implementation.* The individual is in the process of trying to change.

- *Maintenance.* The individual has made the change and is trying hard not to relapse.

The stages of change model can be used in conjunction with models of health belief and behaviour to assess readiness to change and identify important factors that need to be considered in relation to making the change. This is illustrated in the example given below:

- *Pre-contemplation.* At this stage, health promotion is important to draw attention to the need to change and to encourage a set of shared values that will encourage people to want to consider changing their behaviour. The media play an important role in highlighting health issues and raising awareness. Personal advice from health professionals and physiological feedback on personal fitness are important cues to change. The perceived health threat components of the HBM and the attitudes component of the TPB are useful aids in identifying individual beliefs and attitudes that need to be addressed at this stage.
- *Contemplation.* If the individual is thinking about change, the cost–benefit analysis component of the HBM may be helpful to assess potential barriers that might deter them. It might also be useful to use the subjective norm component of the TPB to assess factors likely to influence the individual's intention to change. Health education needs to focus on reinforcing the need for change and helping the individual to set up an action plan.
- *Action planning and implementation.* The perceived behavioural control element of the TPB and barriers component of the HBM are likely to be particularly important in developing and implementing a sustainable plan of action. In the example given above, Mark wanted to change and intended to change, but did not feel sufficiently in control of the barriers to make and maintain the change. Health education can be used to ensure that the individual has the skills to make the change and to recognize and identify ways of overcoming potential barriers.
- *Maintenance.* Maintaining a change in behaviour is often more difficult than making the initial change. For example, relapse rates for those quitting smoking and drinking are high. Health education programmes need to encourage individuals to identify the factors most likely to tempt them to relapse and to plan how to deal with these situations. Social support is particularly important at this stage.

The stages of change model is intuitively attractive and widely used as a basis for cessation of smoking (Riemsma *et al.* 2003). Riemsma reviewed the available research and found little evidence that programmes based on the stage model are more effective than other approaches. However, he suggested that little attention has been given to the rigour of patient assessment. We suggest that using the stages of change model in conjunction with social cognition models such as the HBM and TPB may enhance outcomes (see Courneya *et al.* 2000). Taking the example of Jo's diet, it is clear from an assessment using the health belief model that he is at a stage of pre-contemplation. He is neither intending to change nor contemplating a change. Mark on the other hand, is at the stage of action planning and needs to develop strategies to overcome important barriers.

Self-regulation and health-related behaviour change

Self-regulation implies that people have, or can develop, autonomy, self-control, self-direction and self-discipline (Purdie and McCrindle 2002). These are important assumptions of social cognitive theories. Self-regulation implies that behaviour is purposive and goal-directed, and that motivation comes from the wish to achieve desired goals. It also implies that people are able to anticipate positive and negative outcomes of actions designed to achieve their goals (Bandura 1997). The notion of the self-regulatory system has its origins in systems theory (from which also come the concepts of control, homeostasis and cybernetics). The self-regulatory model assumes that behaviours are all directed towards the achievement of a desired goal (Gollwitzer and Oettingen 2000). Self-regulation depends on feedback through which the individual can appraise and adjust their performance. The amount of effort put into goal achievement is likely to depend on the desirability and achievability of the goal.

Based on these assumptions, it is important to identify an explicit goal, or set of goals, that the individual really wishes to achieve. The problem is that when considering a lifestyle change, people often face competing goals and subgoals. For example, Mark wishes to stay healthy but also enjoys eating unhealthy snacks. Taylor and Gollwitzer (1995) also identified the tendency for people to be unrealistically optimistic in their beliefs about their ability to achieve their goals. We have already considered that they may be poor at anticipating the barriers they are likely to encounter. But Taylor and Gollwitzer suggest that they may also be poor at taking account of competing or conflicting desires, the amount of effort required to overcome habits and social pressures, and the distractions likely to occur. Therefore Gollwitzer and Oettingen (2000) argued that behaviour change requires a goal implementation strategy and not just a goal-directed intention, as proposed in the TPB. It requires that people plan exactly how they will deal with the types of temptation and situational influences we have already discussed.

When Mark developed angina, he needed a plan to avoid the temptation of buying crisps and chocolate. He realized that he also enjoyed the daily chat with the newsagent, who had become a good friend. So he planned to share his problem with his friend and engage his help in buying chewing gum and nuts instead. Meanwhile, he and Janice worked out a lunchtime diet that would satisfy his hunger as well as his dietary needs. This new strategy worked very well. Mark lost weight and started to feel better.

According to Bandura (2000: 316), 'health promotion and risk reduction programs are often structured in ways that are costly, cumbersome and minimally effective'. He asserted that it is impossible to achieve success if the individual has a goal without a plan to achieve it; or if they have a plan without a clearly identified goal. According to Bandura, self-regulation does not rely on will-power, but on having a comprehensive plan. The self-regulatory model does not exclude the models previously discussed, since these may be helpful in assessing readiness for change and identifying potential barriers and resources that need to be incorporated into the implementation plan.

Bandura (2000) drew on behavioural principles to recommend that the individual identifies short-term attainable subgoals to motivate and guide their efforts. The type of programme he recommends is similar to the one outlined by Marks *et al.* (2000); see Chapter 4 and incorporates a range of activities to improve health. Bandura described a computerized distance-directed programme. The achievement of each individually negotiated sub-goal (towards smoking cessation, exercise increase, weight control, stress management) is self-monitored and submitted to the programme director with whom participants are also able to maintain telephone contact for support as necessary. Success depends on having an agreed goal, a set of achievable subgoals, a plan of action, feedback on performance, and availability of support. Bandura (2000) demonstrated how, using a computerized programme, it is possible to oversee the behaviour change of hundreds of participants simultaneously.

Medical help-seeking

The previous sections have focused on beliefs and behaviours associated with primary and secondary prevention. The next sections explore what happens once people have developed symptoms of illness. First it is necessary that people recognize that there is something wrong with them. Then it is essential that they seek help as soon as possible. Cancer and myocardial infarction (MI) are probably the best examples of how delay in seeking medical help can affect the outcome.

Grunefeld *et al.* (2003) surveyed well women about their beliefs and intentions to seek help for breast cancer symptoms, using the theory of planned behaviour. Older women were more likely to express the intention of seeking help than younger women. The inability to recognize breast cancer symptoms predicted delay in all age groups. In addition, for women aged 35–54, lack of perceived behavioural control (not knowing what to expect or what to do) was found to be an important predictor of the intention not to seek help. In women aged over 65 years, negative beliefs about the disabling or disfiguring consequences of having breast cancer was important.

Findings such as these have important implications for health promotion and education. All women need clear information about what to look for and when to seek help, but they also need information about outcomes. The authors suggest that older women might be more concerned about disfigurement if friends or relatives had received surgery at a time when aesthetic outcomes were poor. Providing information about cosmetic outcomes is therefore important.

In the case of MI, delaying the commencement of thrombolytic intervention can have serious adverse effects on outcomes. Yet people often delay calling for help for several hours. Older people may be less likely to summon help because symptoms are less typical or severe. Women may be more likely to delay than men if they view MI as a man's disease. But apart from instances where symptoms are ambiguous, there is little evidence from the literature that lack of knowledge is associated with delay. Similarly, a search for personality factors has not proved useful. But an important reason for delay may be found in social processes of seeking help. For example, a German interview study of post-MI patients (Kentsch *et al.* 2002) found that key factors associated with delay included not wanting to bother anybody, and waiting to ask others for advice.

> When Mark first experienced an attack of angina, he wondered if he might be having a heart attack and was very frightened. It was late afternoon and he was at work. He managed to convince himself that it was probably indigestion and made an excuse to leave early, knowing that Janice would be home. It was Janice who phoned for the ambulance. Fortunately, tests revealed it to be an angina attack and his symptoms responded to treatment. But had it been an MI, his delay could have been fatal.

This scenario is fairly typical. People commonly seek the help, advice and reassurance from others when they feel ill and it is often a family member or friend who prompts help-seeking. This suggests that those who are socially isolated are more likely to get ill and delay seeking help (Chapter 7).

A group identified in the literature as at particular risk of delay in seeking medical help are those with mental health problems. Christiana *et al.* (2000) conducted an international survey of members of patient advocate groups suffering from anxiety disorders and found a median delay of 8 years. Older people were more likely to seek help earlier. An important reason for delay may be the stigmatization of those with a diagnosed mental illness (Chapter 2).

Psychological perspectives on illness

Psychologists in the 1980s found that there are five key questions that people normally want answered when they become ill (Leventhal and Nerenz, 1982; Lau and Hartman 1983).

- *Identity*: what is the name of the disease I have?
- *Consequences*: what will happen to me?
- *Timeline*: what is the duration of the illness?
- *Causes*: why has this happened to me?
- *Cure*: what can be done about it?

Identity refers to a medical label. It is generally very stressful and worrying to be uncertain about what is wrong with you, and patients will often go to great lengths to find a label. It seems a paradox that some patients express relief when given a potentially life-threatening diagnosis such as cancer or multiple sclerosis. A diagnosis validates their illness and their reason for seeking help (see 'Breaking bad news' in Chapter 3). Certain disorders such as back pain and myalgic encephalopathy (ME) may have no definitive diagnostic test and are therefore not acknowledged as 'diseases' by some doctors. It is tempting in such situations for doctors to search for psychological reasons to explain what they believe might be a psychogenic illness. But this can be demoralizing for patients who reject a psychological explanation for their physical symptoms.

The medical model of disease is commonly associated in the public mind with treatment and 'cure'. Yet in reality, relatively few diseases are amenable to cure. Infectious diseases caused by bacteria can often be cured with antibiotics, though resistance is increasingly common. Many 'virus infections' are diagnosed by their symptoms alone and have no cure. Diseases such as cancer are increasingly responsive to drug therapies, though a cure is still some way off. Although medicine is regarded as a science, the causes of some diseases have subsequently been found to be wrong and former treatments to be ineffective. For example, gastric ulcers were until recently believed to be a result of excessive secretion of acid caused by stress (Chapter 7). In fact, feelings of anxiety associated with stomach ulcers were most likely a consequence of physiological discomfort, made worse by the failure of the symptoms to respond to treatment.

Having a diagnosis often (though not always) makes it easier to answer other questions about consequences, time line, causes and cures. But there is no answer to the question 'why me?'. In a British study of beliefs about current and future health, most people strongly rejected the role of chance, fate, or supernatural powers, including God, in influencing their health (Furnham 1994). In contrast, those belonging to the Islamic faith are more likely to attribute disease to 'God's wish' or 'fate' (Baider and De-Nour 1986). This may make it easier to accept situations where there is no cure.

The Illness Perception Questionnaire (IPQ-R; Weinman *et al.* 2004) was designed to assess illness beliefs, based on the dimensions presented above. These include:

- Identity – rating of key symptoms.
- Timeline – is the illness perceived as temporary or permanent?
- Consequences – is the illness perceived to have a major impact on life?
- Illness coherence – does the individual understand their illness?
- Treatment control – does the individual perceive the illness to be controllable or curable?
- Emotional impact – anxiety / depression

Although rather long for use in clinical practice, the IPQ-R is available on the internet and provides a useful example of the types of beliefs that may be amenable to change as a result of a programme to improve coping and symptom management.

Adherence to or concordance with medical advice

Until quite recently, it was assumed patients should be expected to comply with prescribed medical treatments. Non-compliance is costly for patients in terms of their health; for professionals in terms of the frustrations and helplessness caused; and for health services because of wastage and increased demands on health services.

> Compliance has been extensively studied in relation to diabetes. In addition to control over glycaemia, control over blood pressure and lipidaemia are important to reduce long-term adverse health outcomes. Therefore medication and diet are essential aspects of diabetes management. A Canadian study (Toth *et al.* 2003) found that only 10% of its sample met guidelines for glycaemia control. But non-compliance was not restricted to patients. The researchers found that only 22% of diabetic patients were receiving aspirin in line with clinical practice guidelines.

Compliance can also have unfortunate consequences. For example, some people continue to take medication in the face of adverse drug reactions, just because they were told to do so. Donovan and Blake (1992) argued that non-compliance is often a process of reasoned decision-making on the part of the patient, based on a cost–benefit analysis of treatment, while Fogarty (1997) explained non-compliance as reactance against loss of freedom.

Compliance implies obedience to doctor's orders (Chapter 6). This authoritarian and paternalistic perspective was challenged and replaced by the notion of 'adherence'. Adherence entails an agreement between doctor and patient, but still implies that the main agenda is that set by the doctor. Therefore, compliance and adherence both imply varying degrees of coercion, placing the patient in a passive role and discouraging personal control. These issues led Anderson and Funnell (2000) to claim that compliance and adherence are dysfunctional concepts.

The term 'concordance' has more recently been encouraged within health care (Concordance Co-ordinating Group 2000). Concordance implies a shared understanding between health care professional and patient about the nature of the illness, and its treatment and management. The intention is to involve patients as partners in order to ensure that their needs are met.

Sanz (2003) found that when dealing with children with chronic diseases, concordance is required between three partners: doctor, parent and child. Sanz pointed out that the medical consultation frequently involves a two-way conversation between the doctor and parent, while the children plays a passive role. On the other hand, children with asthma or diabetes are expected to play an active role in the management of their disease. This requires the child to play an important part in establishing and agreeing goals and action plans. It also requires that they fully understand the implications of what they are required to do and why.

Partnership involves give and take. Patients need to understand the reasons for and advantages of adhering to a particular course of action. Professionals need to understand the barriers likely to make this difficult. Through partnership, a plan of action or, if necessary, a compromise may then be worked out. In reality, time constraints, the need to use evidence-based treatments, and an unequal power relationship between doctor and patient can mean that coercion is implicit (Ferner 2003). Unequal power relationships are particularly problematic when children are the patients, as illustrated above. However, children can be helped to overcome this.

Igoe (1988, 1991) developed an education programme to improve children's involvement in their own health and health care. In one study, children were asked to draw the medical consultation. They depicted a large doctor, medium-sized mummy and, to one side, a small child, reflecting the interpersonal situation as they saw it. They then received training in what to expect in a medical consultation about themselves, and preparation in how to ask questions. After the programme, their drawings indicated a much more equal relationship between the three partners, as illustrated by the size and position of the three players.

Adherence and health professionals

Discussion of adherence usually refers to patient beliefs and behaviours. However, the health-related beliefs and behaviours of staff are of equal importance to health outcomes. Ley (1997) catalogued activities in which health care professionals had been shown not to comply with standard protocols and procedures. These included observing rules about the administration of drugs, giving adequate patient information, attending professional updates, and adhering to infection control procedures.

Hospital-acquired infection is extremely costly in terms of financial cost and human suffering. One of the most effective ways of reducing it is effective hand-washing, yet compliance by health care professionals appears poor. It is possible to apply the theory of planned behaviour to analyse this issue.

- Do staff believe that failure to wash their hands could have important consequences? Knowledge about the method and frequency of hand-washing is clearly important, but education alone is not sufficient.
- Do staff believe that others who matter believe that they should wash their hands, and how motivated are they to comply with that wish? Infection control is not always accorded highest priority for busy staff. Given the pressures on time, it is always tempting to cut corners. Seeing other staff members cut corners leads people to do the same. But peer pressure can also be used as a force for change.
- Do staff feel able to engage in adequate hand-washing – and if not, why not? Barriers to hand-washing include lack of time and lack of immediately available facilities. One solution to this has been to introduce cleansing hand-rubs at the bedside. The use of rubber gloves is not an appropriate solution because they can increase the sense of invulnerability among staff, while failing to protect patients.

A paediatrician told Anna how bacteria had been eliminated from a neonatal unit. Spot hand cultures were taken from staff. These showed that some members of staff had unacceptable concentrations of bacterial growth. The infection control staff fed back the results to the unit anonymously. This meant that everyone knew that certain people were not washing their hands properly, but did not know who. The next time cultures were taken the results were all clear. This approach appeared to increase self-conscious awareness, and may have made people aware that the eyes of others were on them.

Overall, it should not be assumed that patient behaviour is any different from that of health professionals themselves. Social cognitive theories can be useful for analysing non-compliance in all types of situation.

Self management in chronic disease

This section considers psychological approaches to the management of chronic disease. At the beginning of the twenty-first century, the Department of Health (2001) advocated a new model of care for people with chronic diseases and disorders which they termed the 'expert patient' programme:

> "today's patients with chronic diseases need not be mere recipients of care. They can become key decision-makers in the treatment process. By ensuring that knowledge of their condition is developed to a point

where they are empowered to take some responsibility for its management and work in partnership with their health and social care providers, patients can be given greater control over their lives. Self-management programmes can be specifically designed to reduce the severity of symptoms and improve confidence, resourcefulness and self-efficacy." (DoH 2001: 5)

The purpose of self-management is to preserve or promote health and well-being *in spite of* chronic disease (DoH 2001). Specifically, the aims of self-management are to:

- improve self-efficacy and personal control;
- improve effective symptom management;
- improve activity and function;
- reduce demands on health services in terms of consultations and admissions.

Patients are often informed by doctors that they will have to learn to live with their problem. Drawing on the self-regulatory model discussed earlier in this chapter, this advice is extremely unhelpful unless accompanied by help in developing a goal-directed plan of action. Self-management programmes are designed to achieve just this. Patients are taught ways of controlling their symptoms and believe in their own ability to maintain control over their condition, with professional support. This incorporates principles of cognitive behavioural therapy (Chapter 4). The self-management programme developed by Kate Lorig to help people with rheumatoid arthritis (Lorig *et al.* 1993) was influential in developing the approach recommended by the Department of Health (2001). Lorig's arthritis self-management course demonstrated sustained decreases in pain and depression, increase in perceived self-efficacy and decrease in GP visits (Lorig *et al.* 1993). Self-management reduces costs because it meets patients' needs.

Miller (1992) explained that all of the following aspects need to be considered when developing a self-management strategy:

- maintaining a sense of the 'normal' in daily routines and lifestyle;
- gaining knowledge and skill for symptom management;
- making decisions about treatment;
- using effective coping strategies;
- complying with essential medical regimes;
- dealing with stigma associated with the disorder;
- adjusting to altered social relationships;
- coming to terms with losses associated with the illness;
- maintaining hope.

These reflect much of the contents of this book. Bandura's social learning theory supports the need to learn technical skills, such as the use of inhalers or giving of injections. Modelling and instruction are used to increase self-efficacy in these tasks. Behaviourist principles support the need to identify and reduce avoidance behaviours, reduce risk behaviours and build in treats to reward adherence. Beck's cognitive theory supports the need for positive thinking – focusing on what can be achieved, rather than what cannot be done. Hassles and losses need, where appropriate, to be identified and addressed. Self-regulatory theory supports the need to identify short-term achievable goals as well as longer-term realistic goals to maintain hope. Self-management and cognitive-behavioural programmes have been successfully used to treat rheumatoid arthritis, asthma and diabetes, as well as chronic pain (Chapter 4).

One of the first successful examples of self-management was the programme designed by Thomas Creer to treat childhood asthma (Creer *et al.* 1992). As part of the programme, children were taught to understand their condition and their symptoms, use their inhalers correctly, monitor their own symptoms and learn to recognize early signs of an attack. This enabled them to use their inhaler to prevent or reduce an attack. They rehearsed these skills for implementation at home and at school. The evaluation of the programme identified that the child's locus of control shifted from external to internal, meaning that they felt more control over their lives. However, the researchers noted that parents felt some loss of their parental role, which may need to be addressed.

Asthma self-management programmes have also been developed for adults (see Kotses and Harver 1998). An evaluation by Muntner *et al.* (2001) found that those who declined to participate in their programme had less knowledge about what to do in the event of an attack and less knowledge about the correct use of inhalers. This confirms that those with the greatest need for knowledge and skill may be least likely to attend a self-management programme. It is also worth noting that autonomy and control are not valued equally in all societies. Therefore self-management programmes may fail to cater for the needs of some people from different cultural backgrounds. Nevertheless, nurses and health care professionals in western countries have been at the forefront of the development of self-management programmes.

LeFort *et al.* (1998) adapted Lorig's arthritis self-management course to develop a community-based treatment programme for people with chronic pain in Canada. Significant benefits were decrease in pain and dependency, and increase in vitality, aspects of role functioning, life satisfaction, self-efficacy and resourcefulness (problem-solving coping).

The purpose of self-management and expert patient programmes is to give control to patients. Expert patients are rewarding to work with, but are challenging in terms of their knowledge and may be viewed as a threat by professionals who see themselves as the experts. More recently, health care professionals have gone even further by involving expert patients as peer teachers on self-management programmes.

Peer teaching

Peer teaching in health education has been used in some schools for quite some time, based on the principles of Vygotsky (Chapter 5) and others.

Campbell and McPhail (2002) explored peer teaching in the context of HIV prevention among young people in Africa. They identified that traditional didactic methods of health education seek to change the views and attitudes of single individuals. By contrast, peer education promotes dialogue and argument between peers, as they ask one another questions, exchange anecdotes and comment on one another's experiences and points of view. This provides a forum where peers can weigh up the pros and cons of a range of coping possibilities, using their own terminology and taking account of their own priorities.

Disease-specific self-management group programmes that involve lay teachers or facilitators are becoming increasingly popular. Vygotsky proposed that new knowledge and skills could best be assimilated into people's **schemas** or frames of reference one small step at a time, with help and guidance (chapter 5). Health professionals often find it difficult to understand the mindsets of those who have little medical knowledge. Lay people do not share the same understanding of health and illness and often have quite different goals. Therefore, they are likely to find it easier to learn from people who, like themselves, who have had to learn to cope with a similar illness.

Von Korff *et al.* (1998) conducted a randomized controlled trial to compare the effectiveness of usual care with four sessions of group problem-solving for people with back pain, led by trained lay people. The purpose of the programme was to reduce patient worries, encourage self-care and increase activity levels. Participants in the problem-solving programme reported significantly less worry about back pain and more confidence in self-care. Half of the participants showed a 50% or greater reduction in disability scores at 6 months, compared with 33% among the usual care controls.

The Department of Health (2001) recommended an expansion in user-led self-management programmes provided by patient organizations in partnership with health and social care professionals. At the time of writing, it is too soon to evaluate the outcomes of these initiatives, although a number of systematic reviews are registered as 'in progress' with the Cochrane library. Not all self-management and expert patient programmes are comprehensive in terms of their content. The best programmes are likely to be based on self-regulatory psychological principles outlined above, and need to take account of continuing long-term needs for knowledge, skills and peer support among those with chronic diseases.

Evaluating health outcomes

It is essential when setting up a programme of health education, plan of treatment, or self-management programme to measure its effect on important health outcomes. This section reviews approaches to evaluating outcomes in clinical practice. Based on the self-regulatory model, it is essential that all involved in a programme agree its overall goal or purpose. In other words, what is the intervention intended to achieve? Don Berwick, an American paediatrician well known internationally in the field of quality improvement, emphasized that the main goal of health and social care is to eliminate or reduce human suffering (Berwick 2001).

Margaret developed arthritis in her spine and was experiencing a lot of back and leg pain. The doctor prescribed non-steroidal analgesics that alleviated the pain, but she started getting a lot of indigestion. She loved cooking, but felt too ill to cook or eat. She started to feel quite depressed. The doctor advised her to stop taking the tablets. The pain returned worse than before, but her indigestion subsided. She tried taking other painkillers, but these made her constipated. Eventually, she decided that she would much rather put up with the pain than the side effects of medication. She had a visit from an occupational therapist who recommended a perch stool to use in the kitchen so she could cook and wash up without having to stand. The physiotherapist recommended some exercises that relieved the pain. Although she still had a lot of pain, her sense of well-being was greatly enhanced by these interventions.

Margaret's situation is similar to that is faced by many older people. It illustrates that the goal of relieving pain can sometimes lead to an increase in suffering. Focusing on a goal to reduce suffering requires a more holistic approach, involving the identification of important goals and imaginative solutions. Drawing on the self-regulatory model, it is important when working with individuals to identify personally important and achievable subgoals. Margaret's chief subgoal was to be able independently to prepare and cook meals and wash up. Margaret could achieve her goal in spite of pain, but not in spite of the medication. Others would view their pain differently. Success needs to be measured by the extent to which personally relevant subgoals are achieved. Subgoals in self-management programmes may relate to symptom reduction or management, or to physical or social functioning, or both. The overall aim must be to enhance quality of life, but this must take account of competing or conflicting subgoals.

The World Health Organization (2004b) defines 'quality of life' in terms of 'an individual's perception of their position in life in the context of the culture and value systems in which they live and in relation to their goals, expectations, standards and concerns'. During the 1990s, they set up a collaborative research group to produce an internationally valid measure of quality of life, based on focus groups in 15 centres worldwide (see Skevington *et al.* 1999). The issues identified as contributing to general quality of life are shown in Figure 8.5. Many of them are identical to those identified in Maslow's hierarchy of needs. The main difference is that the group did not choose to present these in a hierarchical order of importance. When applied to people with different problems and priorities, additional issues may need to be added and priorities will vary.

Domain I • Pain and discomfort • Energy and fatigue • Sexual activity • Sleep and rest • Sensory functions	**Domain III** • Mobility • Activities of daily living • Dependence on medication or treatment • Dependence on non-medicinal substances • Communication capacity • Working capacity	**Domain V** • Physical safety and security • Home environment • Work satisfaction • Financial resources • Health and social care: availability and quality • Opportunities for acquiring new information and skills • Participation and opportunities for recreation/leisure • Activities • Physical environments
Domain II • Positive feelings • Thinking, learning, memory and concentration • Self-esteem • Body image and appearance • Negative feelings	**Domain IV** • Personal relationships • Practical social support • Activities as provider/supporter	**Domain VI** • Spirituality, religion and personal beliefs

Figure 8.5 World Health Organization indicators of quality of life (Skevington *et al.* 1999).

Measuring health outcomes

Each disease has specific symptoms and impacts that have important consequences for individual patients. But different patients have different needs. Therefore, using a predetermined set of measurable outcomes may not demonstrate that individual needs have been met. We therefore consider two approaches to measurement: those that are professionally determined and those that accommodate individual needs.

Professionally determined outcome measurement

The evaluation of a self-management programme in clinical practice requires the following:

- Short and simple outcome measures that are relevant, valid and reliable, and capable of demonstrating measurable improvements that are clinically important. Most of these are likely to be based on self-report, which can lead to response bias (Chapter 6).
- Measures need to be multidimensional in order to reflect different aspects of quality of life, for example, improvements in symptoms, physical and social functioning, psychological well-being, and satisfaction.
- Baseline measurements to be established and taken before the programme starts.
- Follow-up measurements to be taken after completion of the programme.

There are two approaches traditionally used by researchers and clinicians to evaluate programme outcomes for research purposes. In the earliest approach, the professionals predict what improvements are likely to be achieved, based on the theoretical predictions on which the programme aim and content are based. These are likely to include increase in well-being and activity. Success is based on statistical probability, but this does not necessarily imply a meaningful result. For example, what does a statistically significant improvement in pain of one point on a scale of 0–100 actually mean?

More recently, the emphasis has moved to include clinically important outcomes. The professionals select the measures, as above, and then work with a team of 'expert patients' or user representatives to determine what would constitute a clinically important improvement on each of the selected measures. In this case, the findings must be both statistically significant and clinically important for the intervention to be judged 'clinically effective'. Most studies now present results in terms of number needed to treat (NNT). NNT refers to the number of patients who need to be treated in order to obtain an agreed level of improvement.

Measurements used by researchers need to facilitate comparisons with the findings of previous studies. Therefore, they usually select measures used in previous studies. This does not always lead to the use of the best instruments. A useful introduction to the measurement of health outcomes, together with comprehensive reviews of a range of health measures, is given by Bowling (1997). There are several global measures of well-being and quality of life, among them the Hospital Anxiety and Depression Scale (HADS) for psychological well-being; the Sense of Coherence Scale (SOC) measuring life satisfaction and meaning; the Short-Form-36 Health Survey Questionnaire (SF36) and Euroquol EQ-5D, which gauge general health status; and the World Health Organization Quality of Life measure (WHO-QOL: see Skevington *et al.* 1999; O'Connell *et al.* 2003) and the Schedule for the Evaluation of Individual Quality of Life (SEIQOL: O'Boyle *et al.* 1993), which are multidimensional measures.

Bowling (2001) also provides a useful review of measures related to a range of specific symptoms and diseases. Symptoms such as pain may be measured using a visual analogue scale (VAS), numerical rating scale (NRS) or verbal rating scale (VRS). It is essential that the measure suits the target population. For example, older people find a six-point VRS easier than visual or numerical systems (Walker 1989) because it is easy to comprehend and can be presented visually or verbally.

An increase in self-efficacy or confidence is a useful indicator of improvement in physical or psychological functioning. There are a variety of disease-specific self-efficacy measures available that are relatively short and simple to use (see Walker 2001), though these tend to prioritize symptom management.

User-led outcome measurement

User-led outcome measurement is more in keeping with the self-regulatory model. Individual patients taking part in the evaluation nominate dimensions they consider to be important in their lives and rate themselves on these dimensions (similar to the repertory grid, Chapter 3). An example used in palliative care is the SEIQOL (O'Boyle *et al.* 1993). Having selected areas that are important to their quality of life, patients rate their current status in each area, and weight the priority given to each, before and after the intervention. The full version of the SEIQOL is reported to be too lengthy and complex for use in clinical practice (Bowling 2001), though a shortened version is being tested for use in clinical settings and is proving popular in cancer and palliative care (Lindblad *et al.* 2002).

A compromise approach is possible. Here, professionals identify certain domains in which improvement is judged to be important (e.g. symptom reduction, increase in mental, social or physical activity, improvement in well-being). Each patient then selects symptoms and activities that are important to them. Success is measured by statistical and/or clinical improvements on each of these dimensions. A good example of this approach to measurement is the freely available (Measure Yourself Medical Outcomes Profile (MYMOP; Paterson 2003), which is simple, quick and easy to use in clinical practice.

After Ted developed chronic heart disease, he was fortunate to join a pilot self-management group involving lay teachers to help improve his quality of life. As part of the evaluation, he completed the MYMOP2 questionnaire (Paterson 2003). Before the programme began, he identified his worst symptom as breathlessness, which he scored 5/6, his difficult activity as gardening (6/6) and he scored his well-being as 4/6 (note that high scores are all negative). He was also asked how many times he had visited his doctor during the last month. One month after the programme finished, he was sent a follow-up questionnaire. This time, he rated his breathlessness as 4/6; his gardening ability as 4/6 and his well-being as 2/6. He had enjoyed the programme and learned some new techniques from staff and 'expert patients'. He felt much less anxious about his condition. As a result, he felt less breathless and more confident to spend time pottering in the garden and greenhouse. The evaluation team were pleased to note that most participants reported fewer visits to their doctor's surgery after the programme. This enabled them to calculate that the cost of putting on the programme was more than balanced by savings to the National Health Service.

Simple tools like this make it easier for health care professionals to establish whether or not interventions are meeting patients' needs.

Summary of key points

- Health and illness are subjective experiences that need to be understood in their social and cultural context.
- Social cognition models, including the health belief model, the theory of planned behaviour and the stages of change model, can be used to assess patient needs and inform health education activities.
- Adherence can be understood using social cognition models and applied to the behaviour of health professionals as well as patients.
- Self-management is based on the principle of self-regulation and involves partnership between health care professionals and service users to promote expert patients.
- Health outcome measures, including quality of life, are important components in the evaluation of health care interventions.

Further reading

Bowling, A. (1997) *Measuring Health*. Buckingham: Open University Press.
Norman, P., Abraham, C. and Conner, M. (eds) (2000) *Understanding and Changing Health Behaviour: From Health Beliefs to Self-Regulation*. Amsterdam: Harwood.

CASE STUDY

- How can health care professionals deal effectively with distress and anger in the immediate situation?
- How can patients and caregivers be encouraged to resolve complex issues through their own actions?

Introduction

For this final chapter, we have selected an actual case study to illustrate how psychology can be applied to patient care. It is based on an encounter that took place in a pain relief clinic and involves multiple problems of the kind that frequently makes nurses, doctors and other health care professionals feel rather helpless. Pseudonyms are used and some details have been changed to protect identities.

The case study is used to illustrate the application of theory to practice and uses an eclectic mix of psychological perspectives contained in this book. However, instead of referencing primary sources of evidence, as normally expected in an academic piece of work, we have indicated where sources that support the analysis can be found in this book. In this way, the case study is used to encourage reading and support further learning.

Case study

The case study focuses on a nurse who worked part-time in a pain clinic assessing new patients. Unusually, the nurse encountered this particular patient just as she was leaving the pain consultant's room.

> Pam was accompanied by her husband, Rob. When the nurse met them in the corridor, Pam was in tears and her husband looked angry.

Non-verbal signs of anger and distress suggested that neither Pam nor Rob felt their needs had been met as a result of the consultation (Chapters 6 and 8). Their distress indicated the need for a helping response (Chapter 6). At that stage, the nurse had no idea what the problem was and decided that the best approach was to listen. Listening helps to establish a therapeutic relationship, and it would provide the nurse with an opportunity to find out what Pam and Rob felt was wrong (Chapter 3). At this time, the nurse had not had the opportunity to look at the medical notes and was not biased by prior expectations (Chapter 2). The nurses's goal for Pam and Rob was to find ways of promoting their well-being (Chapter 8).

> The nurse took Pam and Rob into an empty office. Rob did all the talking, while Pam sat and cried. He explained that Pam had extremely poor circulation. Pam held out her blue hands as he explained that the fingers on her left hand had already been part amputated and those on her right hand caused her excruciating pain most of the time. They had come to the pain clinic to seek relief from the pain, but the doctor had told them that he was unable to help until she gave up smoking. Rob expressed the view that everyone in health care was anti-smoking. He said that Pam had tried hard to give up, but had so many problems that it was unreasonable to expect her to succeed.

The pain was caused by poor circulation. The only treatment available was sympathectomy (cutting the sympathetic nerve supply to the arms) in order to increase the circulation to the hands. But smoking would negate this treatment because nicotine constricts the peripheral blood vessels. The doctor had probably explained this, but it was clear that neither Pam nor Rob had heard or understood it (Chapter 3). They had interpreted the advice to stop smoking as an instruction that required compliance (Chapters 6 and 8). In recommending smoking cessation, the doctor did not appear to have identified an action plan to achieve this (Chapter 8).

> The nurse explained why it was necessary to stop smoking. She explained that the doctor was himself a heavy smoker and would have been sympathetic to Pam's difficulties. She also expressed sympathy with Pam for the difficulties she faced in trying to give up smoking.

The psychology of persuasion suggests that health advice is better received if it appears unprejudiced (Chapter 6). It was clear that Rob felt Pam was being blamed for her lack of will power, rather than being given help to deal with external problems (Chapter 2). It was becoming clear that Pam was under a lot of stress due to her illness and possibly due to other issues, leading to a sense of helplessness and hopelessness. This was possibly compromising her immune response and causing an increased pain response (Chapter 7). Encouraging Pam and Rob to tell their story was likely to reveal useful information for assessment, and might also have therapeutic benefit (Chapter 5).

> Rob explained that he and Pam, both in their early forties, had been married for over twenty years. About ten years ago, Rob discovered that Pam had developed a drink problem. This eventually became so bad that he left her.

Alcohol is often used as an anaesthetic to help people to forget traumatic experiences. It is a means of avoiding reality and reducing distress, and could be classed as a type of emotion-focused coping (Chapter 7). It is maladaptive because it leads to physical health problems, problems with personal relationships and is associated with depression.

> Two years ago, Pam had a stroke that left her with a left-sided weakness and slow in formulating speech. This, Rob explained, was why Pam did not like talking to people. Rob returned home to look after her on the promise that she would give up drinking, which she did.

Rob paused at this point and both he and the nurse expressed admiration for Pam. Alcoholism in women is stigmatized (Chapter 2), and there is a tendency to focus on the previous addiction, rather than the success of stopping.

> Rob went on to explain how he now took care of Pam. He took her breakfast in bed, helped her dress and undress, did all the housework and cooking. He was self-employed and went home at lunchtime to get her a midday meal.

The literature on chronic pain suggests that instrumental support (practical help) can reduce personal control, reinforcing external locus of control (Chapter 4). Having an attentive spouse has been shown to be associated with increased depression in those with chronic pain (Chapter 4) and creates dependence (Chapter 7).

At this stage, Pam and Rob appeared to relax. Possibly they were beginning to feel that their needs were being addressed through the informational and emotional social support they were receiving from the nurse (Chapter 7). The nurse asked Pam to describe her typical day and it became evident that she was able to communicate effectively when she felt more confident.

> Pam described how she watched television all day. She brightened as she said that she looked forward to her husband coming home. She could identify only one programme that she particularly enjoyed and this was a soap that they watched together after Rob and she had supper.

Watching television is a passive coping strategy that provides little by way of distraction from pain (Chapter 7). It became clear that Pam had virtually no positive reinforcement in her life, other than Rob's company and smoking (Chapter 4). It was therefore necessary to find out if there were other things that Pam enjoyed doing.

> Pam described how she had given up her clerical job when their son was born and had not worked since. She went on to describe how she had spent most of her life in children's homes, where she had met Rob. They had one child who was born with a severe mental and physical handicap and died at the age of 6. They had no other children. After the death of their son, Pam became withdrawn and started drinking. It was clear that she had a very low opinion of herself.

Pam chose to focus on her past, highlighting the importance of her biography to her present outlook. This part of her story illustrates that Pam appears to have had little opportunity to develop a secure attachment relationship during her childhood, which might have left her vulnerable to low self-esteem, depression and substance use (Chapter 5). Since marrying Rob, she had experienced a series of serious losses, uncontrollable life events and hassles associated with the death of their son and her subsequent illness (Chapters 5 and 7). She may have turned to alcohol use as a means of regulating her emotions (Chapter 7). This may have further damaged her sense of self-esteem (Chapter 2). Although Rob appears to be a good source of emotional support, Pam is now totally dependent on him and has no control over any aspect of her life. Further, she may fear that Rob might go away again, leaving her with no control and no support at all (Chapter 7). This analysis illustrates a range of reasons that would make Pam vulnerable to anxiety and depression. It also highlights the importance of maintaining Rob's emotional support.

Applying the self-regulatory model (Chapter 8), it was necessary to clarify Pam's main goal. Pam maintained that relief from pain was her main aim.

> The nurse focused on an assessment of Pam's pain. What was the pain like? When was it worst? What did she do to relieve it at present? Was she ever pain-free? Pam described the pain like a constant toothache. She took sustained release morphine and

> was on antidepressants, which helped her to sleep. But her pain
> was not under control. At that point, Rob intervened to point
> out that Pam was usually pain-free when she woke up in the
> morning.

This observation led the nurse to investigate further the pattern of Pam's
pain.

> Rob went on to observe that the pain actually started after she sat up
> in bed and had her first cigarette. Pam nodded agreement.

The identification of pain as an immediate consequence of smoking was
important in identifying negative consequences of smoking that outweigh
the positive consequences (Chapter 8). Smoking serves a number of
important functions (Chapter 4) and it is necessary to compensate for these
if the smoker is to cut down. Therefore it was necessary to identify all the
reasons why Pam smoked.

> Smoking helped to calm Pam's feelings of anxiety, gave her
> something to do, and she enjoyed smoking.

In order to emphasize the negative consequences of smoking, the nurse
asked Pam to keep a pain diary in which she recorded her levels of pain
intensity before and 20 minutes after smoking each cigarette. This 'functional analysis' (Chapter 4) would provide important feedback on the
effects of smoking on her pain and reduce the pleasurable effects of smoking. It was important to emphasize at this point that will power need play
no part in her giving up smoking. As a start, a device for breaking stimulus
control was chosen (Chapter 4).

> The nurse suggested some techniques to reduce smoking. Pam and
> Rob would agree to leave the cigarettes downstairs so that Pam would
> not be able to access them until she was up and dressed. She would
> place a rubber band around the packet and read aloud her special
> message before smoking each cigarette:
>
> This cigarette will cause me a lot of pain.
> This cigarette is making me ill.
> I don't want to smoke this cigarette.

It was then necessary to encourage Pam and Rob to think about alternative ways of filling her time, focusing on things that Pam could do, rather than what she could not do. It was emphasized that active involvement leads to the release of natural endorphins that help to alleviate pain (Chapter 7). It was important to find activities that involved Rob, so as to reassure Pam that he would not leave if she became more independent. Rob was essential to provide emotional support, but needed to provide less practical help unless absolutely necessary (Chapter 7).

> Rob and Pam agreed that it would be possible for Pam to prepare sandwiches for lunch instead of Rob coming in and getting them. Rob would continue to come home at lunchtime to provide company and help to break up the day. When asked about going out, Pam became very defensive. Rob explained that she was embarrassed because people looked at her hands and she found it difficult to speak to strangers.

Stress management is an important part of a smoking cessation programme, particularly as Pam experienced a lot of stress from pain and problematic memories (Chapter 7). It was necessary to find out if Pam could be persuaded to attend group cognitive behavioural therapy (Chapter 4).

> Pam had enjoyed yoga years ago and found it beneficial. But she would not entertain going out of the house, let alone joining a group. Nevertheless, she was willing to try relaxation exercises at home. When asked about hobbies, she admitted that she had been good at crochet and felt that in spite of her hands, she could probably do this again. Rob agreed to buy some thread for her to try. The conversation also led to the possibility of getting a pet.

Any activity that is pleasurable and fills time will help Pam to achieve her goal. A pet is helpful for many reasons. It provides a source of unconditional positive regard (Chapter 1), a sense of purpose, and a source of active occupation.

The interview was coming to a natural end. It had covered a lot of ground and much of it might be forgotten by the time Pam and Rob arrived home, therefore written information was essential (Chapter 3).

> The nurse wrote out a list of key points for Pam and Rob to take home, including their action plan and a contact telephone number for support.

During this interview, the nurse had established a therapeutic relationship of trust, and uncovered reasons for Pam's current state of hopelessness and low self-esteem. She had identified Pam's key motivations, coping strategies, coping resources and barriers. She had negotiated an action plan that included the collection of data that would provide feedback on the achievement of Pam's goal of reducing pain as well as identifying possible causes of pain. The other important outcome indicator was Pam's emotional state, and Rob was asked to keep a record of his wife's daily mood.

> The encounter had taken just under an hour. At the end, Rob and Pam were smiling and thanked the nurse for her time and interest. They made an appointment to share their progress and review the likelihood of having minor surgery to help control the pain. The nurse also gave a telephone number in case they ran into problems.

It may seem unreasonable to devote so long to an individual patient. But time spent on assessment, and negotiating an individual action plan, needs to be considered against the achievement of the long-term therapeutic outcome. Patients, such as Pam, whose perceived needs have not been met usually continue to make a lot of demands on health services. In this case, focusing on pain or smoking without taking account of the context of Pam and Rob's lives was unlikely to lead to therapeutic benefit (Chapter 8).

> Later, as the nurse read through the patient's medical records, she observed a series of negative comments including 'addictive personality'.

Using psychological theory in an informed way avoids stereotypical assumptions associated with the fundamental attribution error (Chapter 2). In this case, the focus on situational factors was empowering for Pam and Rob, since it meant that they could do things to improve their own situation. It also enabled the nurse to work with Pam and Rob towards the overall goal of improving their quality of life (Chapter 8).

Summary of psychological applications

Psychological theories used to inform this case analysis included:

- humanistic psychology (Chapter 1)
- theories of self, self-esteem, prejudice and the fundamental attribution error (Chapter 2)

- memory and information-giving (Chapter 3)
- reinforcement, stimulus control, self-efficacy and cognitive-behavioural principles applied to smoking cessation (Chapter 4)
- loss (Chapter 5)
- interpersonal interactions (Chapter 6)
- stress, coping and control (Chapter 7)
- principles of health education and self-management in chronic disease; and quality of life (Chapter 8).

Summary of key issues

- Distress and anger are best dealt with by listening.
- The presenting problem (e.g. pain or smoking) is rarely the only cause of distress.
- It is important to focus action on the patient's priorities.
- It is necessary to take account of patient's preferences and barriers when negotiating an action plan.
- It is important to ask the patient to collect some simple data that will demonstrate progress.

Further reading

Carter, B. (ed.) (1998) *Perspectives on Pain: Mapping the Territory*. London: Arnold *Journal of Nursing Management* (2004, June) special issue on pain.
Wall, P. (1999) *Pain: The Science of Suffering*. London: Weidenfeld and Nicolson.

GLOSSARY

Active versus passive coping: doing something versus doing nothing when faced with a problem.

Adaptation: a process of change that achieves a desired outcome or has survival value.

Anxiety: a state of emotional and physiological arousal associated with perceptions of threat or lack of control.

Appraisal: thought processes used to evaluate a potential stressor (from Lazarus 1966).

Approach/avoidance: ways of coping with problems, either by confronting them (approach) or avoiding them.

Attachment: a strong emotional bond between two people that elicits caring behaviours.

Attribution theory: from social psychology, a theory of how people make inferences about the causes of behaviour.

Avoidance: behaviours associated with ignoring the existence of problems and any negative consequences.

Behaviourism: an approach to psychology that proposes that all behaviour is determined by its antecedents (cues) and its consequences.

Behaviourist, behavioural: based on the principles of behaviourism.

Bereavement: a perception of loss caused by death.

Biopsychosocial: an approach that views biological, psychological and social systems in combination, rather than separately.

Bipolar: refers to a scale of measure that has a positive and negative pole (e.g. a Likert scale).

Bonding: the formation of a strong attachment relationship.

Burnout: a response to stress in the caring professions that leads to feelings of emotional exhaustion and depersonalizing behaviours towards patients.

Catharsis: a term from psychoanalysis used to describe the therapeutic release of negative emotions.

Classical conditioning: from behaviourism, a simple form of associative learning in which reflex behaviours come under the unconscious control of an external stimulus.

Cognition: thought processes, including perception, memory and information processing.

Cognitive dissonance: a state of emotional tension created by two inconsistent beliefs, or between an incompatibility between the individual's beliefs and their behaviour (from Festinger 1957).

Cognitive behavioural therapy: a structured therapy based on principles from behavioural and cognitive psychology.

Compliance: actions undertaken in accordance with the instructions of others.

Conditioning: a process by which simple associative learning takes place.

Conformity: the tendency for perceptions, attitudes and behaviours to mirror those of the powerful others, or the majority, in social situations.

Coping: ways of dealing with problems.

Coping strategies: conscious methods of dealing with problems.

Daily hassles: minor events that disrupt or interrupt daily routines.

Decentre: the ability to see or feel things from the point of view of another person.

Defence mechanisms: from psychoanalysis, the term used to describe unconscious processes that are assumed to defend the ego from unmanageable threats and anxiety.

Denial: from psychoanalysis, a defence mechanism in which the individual refuses to accept the reality of a situation.

Depersonalization: the treatment of an individual as an object, rather than a person.

Depression: a state of hopelessness and helplessness.

Eclectic: in psychotherapy, a mix of psychological approaches drawn from different schools of thought.

Ego: in psychoanalysis, the part of the mind concerned with conscious self-regulation.

Egocentrism: the inability to see or feel things from the point of view of another individual.

Empiricism: a philosophical belief that all knowledge is gained from experience (the opposite of nativism).

Emotion-focused coping: a form of coping that is intended to relieve unpleasant emotions such as anxiety or fear.

Emotional support: helping people to feel loved, cared for and valued.

Fight or flight response: state of immediate readiness for action, stimulated by a perception of threat (from Cannon 1932).

Functional analysis: from behaviourism, a systematic analysis of cues and consequences that influence behaviour.

Fundamental attribution error: a pervasive tendency to blame people for their own problems or mistakes, rather than looking for situational causes.

Generalized/generalizable: Implies that findings from a sample, or situation, are applicable to the whole population, or to all situations.

Grief: the emotional response to feelings of loss.

Groupthink: group interaction that can lead to erroneous beliefs in the correctness of group decisions (from Janis 1982).

Habit, habitual: a routine pattern of behaviour, not subject to conscious awareness.

Health behaviour: a behaviour directed towards achieving a health goal.

Health-related behaviour: a behaviour that has an impact on health, but is not necessarily directed towards achieving a health goal.

Homeostasis: process by which physiological systems are maintained in a state of balance.

Hypothesis: a prediction that a particular action will lead to a particular outcome.

Iatrogenesis: medically induced illness.

Illness behaviour: behavioural responses to illness that include signalling the need for help.

Inductive: a process of generating theory from observational data.

Informational support: giving advice or information to enhance well-being.

Instrumental support: practical or tangible help.

Introspection: examination of one's own mental experiences.

Learned helplessness: a state of depression caused by perceived uncontrollability and associated with cognitive, motivational and behavioural deficits (from Seligman 1975).

Life events: events involving loss or change that require major adjustment or adaptation.

Likert scale: a measure of agreement versus disagreement that is scaled for the purpose of statistical analysis, e.g.

Strongly agree   Agree   Neutral   Disagree   Strongly disagree

Locus of control: a set of beliefs about internal (personal) or external (other or chance) responsibility for achieving a desired outcome (from Rotter 1966).

Loss: an unpleasant experience caused by separation from a loved person or object.

Maladaptation: responses to change that lead to adverse outcomes or unintended consequences.

Mnemonic: a technique of visual or verbal association used to improve memory for facts.

Modelling: the learning of new skills by observing and copying others (from Bandura 1977a).

Mourning: the behavioural expression of grief, shaped by cultural expectations.

Narrative psychology: psychology based on the belief that our biographical stories constitute our sense of self.

Narrative therapy: therapy that uses therapeutic writing or verbal story telling, with or without the presence of a therapist.

Nativism: a philosophical belief that humans are born with unique abilities to organize knowledge and respond to their environment.

Non-verbal communication: communication by facial expression and body movement.

Normative: in social psychology, social influences to conform.

Operant conditioning: learning by which voluntary behaviours and activities are brought under the control of external stimuli.

Phenomenology: a philosophical doctrine that advocates the study of subjective or 'lived' experience.

Placebo: an inert substance that elicits an expectation of an effect and leads to physiological change.

Placebo response: physiological or psychological change brought about by expectation.

Post hoc: refers to an explanation given after the event (opposite of a priori).

Primacy effect: information given first is remembered best.

Primary appraisal: cognitive process by which the individual determines if there is a threat (from Lazarus 1966).

Problem-focused coping: a response to stress that focuses on resolving the problem.

Psychoanalysis: a method of investigation, theory of mind, and form of treatment invented by Sigmund Freud.

Psychodynamic: refers to psychological systems that emphasize processes of development and change across the lifespan.

Psychogenic: a disease that has a psychological origin.

Psychoneuroimmunology: study of psychological factors that affect the immune system.

Psychosocial: an approach that views psychological and social systems in combination, rather than separately.

Psychosomatic: a disease that has a psychological component, as cause or effect.

Punishment: in behaviourism, an intervention that decreases the likelihood that the target behaviour will occur.

Randomized controlled trial: a research method used to test a new intervention; attempts to control for effects not attributable to the intervention by random allocation to a comparable alternative treatment.

Random: chance occurrence.

Recency effect: information given last is remembered best.

Reference group: a group of people who share desired attributes and goals.

Reinforcement: in behaviourism, an intervention that increases the likelihood that the target behaviour will occur.

Reliablity: when applied to a psychological measurement tool, consistency in producing the same result on separate occasions in similar circumstances.

Repertory grid: a method used to measure the self concept (from Kelly 1955).

Repression: from psychoanalysis, a defence mechanism that suppresses memories that cause anxiety.

Rogerian counselling: based on the work of Carl Rogers, non-directive client-centred therapy provided in an atmosphere of 'unconditional positive regard'.

Schedule of reinforcement: from behaviourism, the frequency or regularity by which reinforcement is received.

Schema: mental representations that inform understanding.

Secondary appraisal: cognitive process by which the individual determines what to do about a perceived threat (from Lazarus 1966).

Self: Personal identity.

Self-actualization: from humanistic psychology, a process of personal growth, or the pinnacle of achievement.

Self-efficacy: belief on one's ability to achieve a desired outcome (from Bandura 1977b).

Self-esteem: feeling good about oneself.

Self-management: learning to deal with an illness and its consequences through one's own actions.

Self-regulation: conscious efforts to achieve a desired goal in a changing environment.

Semantic differential scale: bipolar measure using a five- or seven-point scale, e.g.

Happy |_|_|_|_|_|_| Sad

Sense of coherence: the feeling that one's life is meaningful, from Antonovsky (1985).

Social cognition: study of thought processes in the context of the social environment in which they arise.

Social cognitive theory: theories of how individuals make decisions in social situations.

Social norm: expected standards of belief or behaviour determined by one's social or cultural reference group.

Social support: actions that impact on the well-being of others.

Stigma: distinguishing features that have a negative impact on the attitudes of others (from Goffman 1963).

Stimulus: from behavioural psychology, an internal or external event or change that alerts attention and precipitates arousal.

Stimulus control: from behavioural psychology, the automatic triggering of a response by an external event or situational cue.

Stressor: an internal of external event that is perceived as a potential cause of threat or harm.

Tangible support: see instrumental support.

Threat: any event that potentially threatens physical or psychological well-being.

Unconditional positive regard: from humanistic psychology, esteem that is freely given, regardless of the behaviour or demeanour of the other.

Validity: when applied to a psychological measure, the extent to which it measures what it is intended to measure, and not something else.

REFERENCES

Abrams, D. and Hogg, M.A. (2004) Collective identity: group membership and self-conception. In M.B. Brewer and M. Hewstone (eds) *Self and Social Identity*. Oxford: Blackwell, pp. 147–81.

Ainsworth, M.D.S., Blehar, M.C., Waters, E. and Wall, S. (1978) *Patterns of Attachment*. Hillsdale, NJ: Lawrence Erlbaum Associates.

Ajzen, I. (1988) *Attitudes, Personality and Behaviour*. Milton Keynes: Open University Press.

Ajzen, I. (1991) The theory of planned behavior. *Organizational Behavior and Human Decision Processes*, 50: 179–211.

Ajzen, I. and Fishbein, M. (1980) *Understanding Attitudes and Predicting Social Behavior*. Englewood Cliffs, NJ: Prentice Hall.

Al-Ghazal, S.K., Fallowfeld, L. and Blamey, R.W. (2000) Comparison of psychological aspects and patient satisfaction following breast conserving surgery, simple mastectomy and breast reconstruction. *European Journal of Cancer*, 36: 1938–43.

American Psychiatric Association (2000) *Diagnostic and Statistical Manual of Mental Disorders: DSM-IV®-TR*, 4th edition. Washington, DC: American Psychiatric Association.

Anderson, M.C. (2003) Rethinking interference theory: Executive control and the mechanisms of forgetting. *Journal of Memory and Language*, 9(4): 415–45.

Anderson, R.M. and Funnell, M.M. (2000) Compliance and adherence are dysfunctional concepts in diabetes care. *Diabetes Educator*, 26(4): 597–604.

Antonovsky, A. (1985) *Health, Stress and Coping*. San Francisco: Jossey-Bass.

Armitage, C.J. and Conner, M. (2001) Efficacy of the theory of planned behaviour: A meta-analytic review. *British Journal of Social Psychology*, 40(4): 471–99.

Aronson, E. (1988) *The social animal*, 5th edition. New York: W.H. Freeman.

Asbring, P. (2001) Chronic illness – a disruption in life: identity-transformation among women with chronic fatigue syndrome and fibromyalgia. *Journal of Advanced Nursing*, 34(3): 312–19.

Baider L. and De-Nour A.K. (1986) The meaning of a disease: An exploratory study of Moslem Arab women after a mastectomy. *Journal of Psychosocial Oncology*, 4(4): 1–13.

Bandolier (2004) The Oxford pain internet site. http://www.jr2.ox.ac.uk/bandolier/booth/painpag/

Bandura, A. (1977a) *Social Learning Theory*. Englewood Cliffs, NJ: Prentice Hall.

Bandura, A. (1977b) Self-efficacy: Towards a unifying theory of behavioural change. *Psychological Review*, 84(2): 191–215.

Bandura, A. (1997) *Self-efficacy: The Exercise of Control*. New York: W.H. Freeman.

Bandura, A. (2000) Health promotion from the perspective of social cognitive theory. In P. Norman, C. Abraham and M. Conner (eds) *Understanding and Changing Health Behaviour: From Health Beliefs to Self-regulation*. Amsterdam: Harwood, pp. 299–342.

Bandura, A., Ross, D. and Ross, S.A. (1961) Transmission of aggression through imitation of aggressive models. *Journal of Abnormal and Social Psychology*, 63: 575–82.

Baumrind, D. (1967) Child care practices anteceding three patterns of preschool behaviour. *Genetic Psychology Monographs*, 75: 43–8.

Baumrind, D. (1971) Current patterns of parental authority. *Developmental Psychology Monograph, Part 2*, 4(1), 1–103.

Baumrind, D. (1991) The influence of parenting style on adolescent competence and substance use. *Journal of Early Adolescence*, 11(1): 56–95.

Beck, A.T. (1976) *Cognitive Therapy and the Emotional Disorders*. Harmondsworth: Penguin.

Beck, A.T., Steer, R.A. and Brown G.K. (1997) *Beck Depression Inventory – II*. London: Psychological Corporation.

Becker, M.H. and Maiman, L.A. (1975) Sociobehavioural determinants of compliance with health and medical care recommendations. *Medical Care*, 13: 10–24.

Benner, P. and Wrubel, J. (1989) *The Primacy of Caring: Stress and Coping in Health and Illness*. Menlo Park, CA: Addison-Wesley.

Berwick, D. (2001) Agenda for improvement in health services for the third millennium. Plenary paper given at 6th European Conference on Quality Improvement in Health Care, Bologna, April.

Bibace, R. and Walsh, M. (1981) Children's conceptions of illness. In R. Bibace and M. Walsh (eds) *Children's Concepts of Health, Illness and Bodily Function*. San Francisco: Jossey-Bass.

Blaxter, M. (1990) *Health and Lifestyles*. London: Tavistock/Routledge.

Bohlmeijer, E., Smit, F. and Cuijpers, P. (2003) Effects of reminiscence and life review on late-life depression: A meta-analysis. *International Journal of Geriatric Psychiatry*, 18(12): 1088–94.

Borkenau, P., Riemann, R., Angleitner, A. and Spinath, F.M. (2001) Genetic and environmental influences on observed personality: Evidence from the German observational study of adult twins. *Journal of Personality and Social Psychology*, 80(4): 655–68.

Bowers, K.S. (1968) Pain anxiety and perceived control. *Journal of Consulting and Clinical Psychology*, 32(5): 596–602.

Bowlby, J. (1969) *Attachment and loss: Vol. 1. Attachment*. London: Hogarth Press.

Bowling, A. (1997) *Measuring health*, 2nd edition. Buckingham: Open University Press.

Bowling, A. (2001) *Measuring disease*, 2nd edition. Buckingham: Open University Press.

Brehm, S.S., Kassin, S.M. and Fein, S. (2002) *Social Psychology*, 5th edition. Boston: Houghton Mifflin.

Briner, R. (1994) Stress: The creation of a modern myth. Paper presented at the Annual Conference of the British Psychological Society, Brighton, March.

Brissette, I., Scheier, M.F. and Carver, C.S. (2002) The role of optimism in social network development, coping, and psychological adjustment during a life transition. *Journal of Personality and Social Psychology*, 82(1): 102–11.

Bruner, J.S. (1983) *Child's Talk: Learning to Use Language*. Oxford: Oxford University Press.

Bury, M. (1982) Chronic illness as biographical disruption. *Sociology of Health and Illness*, 4: 167–82.

Butler, R.N. (1974) Successful aging and the role of the life review. *Journal of the American Geriatrics Society*, 22(12): 529–35.

Campbell, C. and MacPhail, C. (2002) Peer education, gender and the development of critical consciousness: Participatory HIV prevention by South African youth. *Social Science and Medicine*, 55(2): 331–45.

Cannon, B. (1932) *The Wisdom of the Body*. New York: Norton.

Carman, M.B. (1997) The psychology of normal aging. *Psychiatric Clinics of North America*, 20(1): 15–24.

Christiana, J.M., Gilman, S.E., Guardino, M., Mickelson, K., Morselli, P.L., Olfson, M. and Kessler R.C. (2000) Duration between onset and time of obtaining initial treatment among people with anxiety and mood disorders: An international survey of members of mental health patient advocate groups. *Psychological Medicine*, 30(3): 693–703.

Clare, L., Woods, R.T., Moniz Cook, E.D., Orrell, M. and Spector A. (2003) Cognitive rehabilitation and cognitive training for early-stage Alzheimer's disease and vascular dementia (Cochrane Review). In *The Cochrane Library* 4. Chichester: Wiley

Clark, P. (2001) Narrative gerontology in clinical practice: Current applications and future prospects. In G. Kenyon, P. Clark and B. de Vries (eds) *Narrative Gerontology: Theory, Research, and Practice*. New York: Springer.

Cobb, S. (1976) Social support as a moderator of life stress. *Psychosomatic Medicine*, 38(5): 300–14.

Cohen, D.A., Richardson, J. and Labree, L. (1994) Parenting behaviors and the onset of smoking and alcohol use: A longitudinal study. *Pediatrics*, 94(3): 368–75.

Cohen, F., Kearney, K.A., Zegans, L.S., Kemeny, M.E., Neuhaus, J.M. and Stites, D.P. (1999) Differential immune system changes with acute and persistent stress for optimists vs pessimists. *Brain, Behaviour and Immunity*, 13: 155–74.

Coleman, L.M. and Ingham, R. (1999) Contraception: how can we encourage more discussion between partners? *Health Education Research* 14(6): 741–50.

Coleman, P.G. (1999) Creating a life story: The task of reconciliation. *The Gerontologist*, 39(2): 133–9.

Concordance Co-ordinating Group (2000) *Concordance – Partnership in Medicine Taking, information pack*. London: Royal Pharmaceutical Society of Great Britain.

Conner, M. and Norman, P. (1995) The role of social cognition in health behaviours. In M. Conner and P. Norman (eds) *Predicting Health Behaviour: Research and Practice with Social Cognition Models*. Buckingham: Open University Press.

Coopersmith, S. (1967) *The Antecedents of Self-esteem*. San Francisco: W.H. Freeman.

Coull, F. (2003) Personal story offers insight into living with facial disfigurement. *Journal of Wound Care*, 12(7): 254–8.

Costa, P.T. and McCrae, R.R. (1992) The five-factor model of personality and its relevance to personality disorders. *Journal of Personality Disorders*, 6(4): 343–59.

Courneya, K.S., Nigg, C.R. and Estabrooks, P.I.A. (2000) Relationships among the theory of planned behaviour, stages of change and exercise behaviour in older persons over a three year period. In P. Norman, C. Abraham and M. Conner (eds) *Understanding and Changing Health Behaviour*. Amsterdam: Harwood, pp. 189–206.

Craig, K.D. (2004) Social communication of pain enhances protective functions: a comment on Deyo, Prkachin and Mercer (2004). *Pain*, 107: 5–6.

Creer, T.L., Stein, R.E., Rappaport, L. and Lewis, C. (1992) Behavioural consequences of illness: Childhood asthma as a model. *Pediatrics*, 90(5): 808–15.

Crombez, G., Vlaeyen, J.W.S., Heuts, P.H.T.G. and Lysens, R. (1999) Pain-related fear is more disabling than pain itself: evidence on the role of pain-related fear in chronic back pain disability. *Pain*, 80: 329–39.

Crossley, M. (2003) 'Let me explain': Narrative emplotment and one patient's experience of oral cancer. *Social Science and Medicine*, 56: 439–48.

Crowne, D.P. and Marlowe, D. (1960) A new scale of social desirability independent of psychopathology. *Journal of Consulting Psychology*, 24: 349–54.

Cumming, E. and Henry, W.E. (1961) *Growing Old: The Process of Disengagement*. New York: Basic Books.

Damon, W. (1983) *Social and Personality Development: Infancy through Adolescence*. New York: W.W. Norton.

De Beni, R. and Palladino, P. (2004) Decline in working memory updating through ageing: Intrusion error analyses. *Memory*, 12(1): 75–89

de Melker, R.A., Touw-Otten, F.W. and Kuyvenhoven, M.M. (1997) Transcultural differences in illness behaviour and clinical outcome: An underestimated aspect of general practice? *Family Practice*, 14(6): 472–7.

Department of Health (1999) *Saving Lives: Our Healthier Nation*. London: Department of Health.

Department of Health (2001) The expert patient: a new approach to chronic disease management for the 21st century. London: Department of Health.

DiClemente, C.C. (1993) Changing addictive behaviours: A process perspective. *Current Directions in Psychological Science*, 2: 101–6.

Dolbier, C.L., Cocke, R.R., Leiferman, J.A., Steinhardt, M.A., Schapiro, S.J. *et al.* (2001) Differences in functional immune responses of high versus low hardy healthy individuals. *Journal of Behavioral Medicine*, 24(3): 219–229.

Donaldson, M. (1990) *Children's Minds*. Glasgow: Fontana.

Donovan, J.L. and Blake, D.R. (1992) Patient non-compliance: Deviance or reasoned decision-making? *Social Science and Medicine*, 34(5): 507–13.

Earnst, K.S., Marson, D.C. and Harrell, L.E. (2000) Cognitive models of physicians' legal standard and personal judgements of competency in patients with Alzheimer's disease. *Journal of the American Geriatrics Society*, 48(8): 919–27.

Ehlers, A. and Clark, D.M. (2000) A cognitive model of post-traumatic stress disorder. *Behaviour Research and Therapy*, 38(4): 319–45.

Eisenberg, L. (1977) Disease and illness. Distinctions between professional and popular ideas of sickness. *Cultural Medical Psychiatry*, 1(1): 9–23.

Eiser, C. and Patterson, D. (1983) 'Slugs and snails and puppy-dog tails' – children's ideas about the inside of their bodies. *Child: Care, Health and Development*, 9: 233–40.

Eiser, J.R. and Gentle, P. (1989) Health behaviour and attitudes to publicity campaigns for health promotion. *Psychology and Health*, 3: 111–20.

Erikson, E.H. (1980) *Identity and the Life Cycle*. New York: Norton.

Esterling, B.A., L'Abate, L., Murray, E.J. and Pennebaker, J.W. (1999) Empirical foundations for writing in prevention and psychotherapy: Mental and physical health outcomes. *Clinical Psychology Review*, 19(1): 79–96.

Evans, A. (1994) Anticipatory grief: a theoretical challenge. *Palliative Medicine*, 8: 159–65.

Falkner, T.M. and de Luce, J. (1992) A view from antiquity: Greece, Rome and elders. In T.R. Cole, D. van Tussel and R. Kastenbaum (eds) *Handbook of the Humanities and Aging*. New York: Springer, pp. 3–39

Fallowfield, L.J., Jenkins, V.A. and Beveridge, H.A. (2002) Truth may hurt but deceit hurts more: Communication in palliative care. *Palliative Medicine*, 16(4): 297–303.

Ferner, R.E. (2003) Is concordance the primrose path to health? *British Medical Journal*, 327(7419): 821–2.

Festinger, L. (1954) A theory of social comparison. *Human Relations*, 7: 117–40.

Festinger, L. (1957) *A Theory of Cognitive Dissonance*. Stanford, CA: Stanford University Press.

Flor, H., Kerns, R.D. and Turk, D.C. (1987) The role of spouse reinforcement, perceived pain and activity levels of chronic pain patients. *Journal of Psychosomatic Research*, 31: 251–9.

Fogarty, J.S. (1997) Reactance theory and patient noncompliance. *Social Science and Medicine*, 45(8): 1277–88.

Folkman, S. and Lazarus, R.S. (1991) The concept of coping. In A. Monat and R.S. Lazarus (eds), *Stress and Coping: An Anthology*, 3rd edition. New York: Columbia University Press, pp. 207–27.

Folkman, S. and Lazarus, R.S. (2003) Ways of Coping Questionnaire (WAYS). http://www.mindgarden.com/Assessments/Info/waysinfo.htm

Folstein, M.F., Folstein, S.E. and McHugh, P.R. (1975) Mini Mental State. *Journal of Psychosomatic Research*, 12: 196–8.

Fordyce, W.E. (1982) A behavioural perspective on chronic pain. *British Journal of Clinical Psychology*, 21: 313–20.

Fox, N.A. and Card, J.A. (1999) Psychophysiological measures in the study of attachment. In J. Cassidy and P.R. Shaver, *Handbook of Attachment: Theory, Research and Clinical Applications*. New York: Guilford Press, pp. 226–48.

Frank, A.W. (1995) *The Wounded Storyteller: Body, Illness and Ethics*. Chicago: University of Chicago Press

Friedman, M. and Rosenman, R.H. (1974) *Type A Behaviour and Your Heart*. New York: Knopf.

Friedman, H.S. (2000) Long-term relations of personality and health: Dynamisms, mechanisms, tropisms. *Journal of Personality*, 68(6): 1089–1107.

Furnham, A. (1994) Explaining health and illness: Lay perceptions on current and future health, the causes of illness, and the nature of recovery. *Social Science and Medicine*, 39(5): 715–25.

Galvin, K.T. (1992) A critical review of the health belief model in relation to cigarette smoking behaviour. *Journal of Clinical Nursing*, 1(1): 13–18.

Garcia, J., Ervin, F.R. and Koelling, R.A. (1966) Learning with prolonged delay to reinforcement. *Psychonomic Science*, 5(3): 121–2.

Gergen, K.J. and Gergen, M.M. (1997) Narratives of the self. In L.P. Hinchman and S.K. Hinchman (eds). *Memory, Identity, Community: The Idea of Narrative in the Human Sciences*. New York: State University of New York Press, pp. 161–84.

Goffman, E. (1959) *The Presentation of Self in Everyday Life*. London: Penguin.

Goffman, E. (1963) *Stigma: Notes on the Management of Spoiled Identity*. Harmondsworth: Penguin.

Gollwitzer, P.M. and Oettingen, G. (2000) The emergence and implementation of health goals. In P. Norman, C. Abraham and M. Conner (eds) *Understanding and Changing Health Behaviour*. Amsterdam: Harwood, pp. 229–60.

Goodwin, R.D., Hoven, C.W., Lyons, J.S. and Stein, M.B. (2002) Mental health service utilization in the United States. The role of personality factors. *Social Psychiatry and Psychiatric Epidemiology*, 37(12): 561–6.

Graham, H. (1993) *Hardship and Health in Women's Lives*. New York: Harvester Wheatsheaf.

Griffin, J.M., Fuhrer, R., Stansfeld, S.A. and Marmot, M. (2002) The importance of low control at work and home on depression and anxiety: Do these effects vary by gender and social class? *Social Science and Medicine*, 54(5): 783–98.

Griffin, K.W., Botvin, G.J., Scheier, L.M., Diaz, T. and Miller, N.L. (2000) Parenting practices as predictors of substance use, delinquency, and aggression among urban minority youth: Moderating effects of family structure and gender. *Psychology of Addictive Behaviors*, 14(2): 174–84.

Grunfeld, E.A., Hunter, M.S., Ramirez, A.J. and Richards, M.A. (2003) Perceptions of breast cancer across the lifespan. *Journal of Psychosomatic Research*, 54(2): 141–6.

Haight, B.K. and Olson, M. (1989) Teaching home health aides the use of life review. *Journal of Nursing Staff Development*, 5(1): 11–16.

Hall, S., Abramsky, L. and Marteau, T.M. (2003) Health professionals' reports of information given to parents following the prenatal diagnosis of sex chromosome anomalies and outcomes of pregnancies: a pilot study. *Prenatal Diagnosis*, 23(7): 535–8.

Härkäpää, K., Järvikoski A., Mellin G., Hurri H., Luoma J. (1991) Health locus of control beliefs and psychological distress as predictors for treatment outcome in low-back pain patients: results of a 3-month follow-up of a controlled intervention study. *Pain*, 46: 35–41.

Harlow, H.F. (1959) Love in infant monkeys. *Scientific American*, 200: 68–74.

Havighurst, R.J., Neugarten, B.L. and Tobin, S.S. (1968) Disengagement and patterns of ageing. In B.L. Neugarten (ed.) *Middle Age and Ageing*. Chicago: University of Chicago Press.

Hazan, C. and Zeifman, D. (1999) Pair bonds as attachments: Evaluating the evidence. In J. Cassidy and P.R. Shaver (eds) *Handbook of Attachment: Theory, Research and Clinical Applications*. New York: Guilford Press pp. 336–54.

Helson, R., Jones, C. and Kwan, V.S.Y. (2002) Personality change over 40 years of adulthood: Hierarchical linear modeling analyses of two longitudinal samples. *Journal of Personality and Social Psychology*, 83(3): 752–66.

Hewison, D. (1997) Coping with loss of ability: 'Good grief' or episodic stress responses? *Social Science and Medicine*, 44(8): 1129–39.

Hewstone, M. (1989) *Causal Attribution: From Cognitive Processes to Collective Beliefs.* Oxford: Blackwell.

Hobfoll, S.E. (1988) *The Ecology of Stress.* New York: Hemisphere.

Hofling, C.K., Brotzman, E., Dalrymple, S., Graves, N. and Pierce, C.M. (1966) An experimental study in nurse–physician relationships. *Journal of Nervous and Mental Disease.* 143(2):171–80

Hogbin, B. and Fallowfield, L. (1989) Getting it taped: the 'bad news' consultation with cancer patients. *British Journal of Hospital Medicine*, 41(4): 330–3.

Holmes, T.H. and Rahe, R.H. (1967) The Social Readjustment Rating Scale. *Journal of Psychsomatic Research*, 11: 213–18.

Houston, V. and Bull, R. (1994) Do people avoid sitting next to someone who is facially disfigured? *European Journal of Social Psychology*, 24(2): 279–284.

Hunt, S.M. and Martin, C.J. (1988) Health-related behavioural change – a test of a new model. *Psychology and Health*, 2: 209–30.

Igoe, J.B. (1988) Healthy long-term attitudes on personal health can be developed in school-age children. *Pediatrician*, 15(3): 127–36.

Igoe, J.B. (1991) Empowerment of children and youth for consumer self-care. *American Journal of Health Promotion*, 6(1): 55–64.

Ingham, R. (1993) Old bodies in older clothes. *Health Psychology Update*, 14: 31–6.

Janis, I.L. (1982) *Groupthink: Psychological Studies of Policy Decisions and Fiascos*, 2nd edition. Boston: Houghton Mifflin.

Janssen, C.G., Schuengel, C. and Stolk, J. (2002) Understanding challenging behaviour in people with severe and profound intellectual disability: a stress-attachment model. *Journal of Intellectual Disability Research*, 46(6): 445–53.

Janz N. and Becker M.H. (1984) The health belief model: a decade later. *Health Education Quarterly*, 11: 1–47.

Johnson, M. and Webb, C. (1995) Rediscovering the unpopular patients: the concept of social judgement. *Journal of Advanced Nursing*, 21(3): 466–74.

Jordan, J.R. and Neimeyer, R.A. (2003) Does grief counseling work? *Death Studies*, 27(9): 765–86.

Keenan, T. (2002) *An Introduction to Child Development.* London: Sage.

Keijsers, G.P., Schaap, C.P. and Hoogduin, C.A. (2000) The impact of interpersonal patient and therapist behavior on outcome in cognitive-behavior therapy. A review of empirical studies. *Behavior Modification*, 24(2): 264–97.

Kelly, G.A. (1955) *A Theory of Personality: The Psychology of Personal Constructs.* New York: W.W. Norton.

Kelly, P. (1998) Loss experienced in chronic pain and illness. In J.H. Harvey (ed.) *Perspectives on Loss: A Sourcebook.* Philadelphia: Brunner Mazel.

Kentsch, M., Rodemerk, U., Müller-Esch, G., Schnoor, U., Münzel, T., Ittel, T.-H. and Mitusch, R. (2002) Emotional attitudes toward symptoms and inadequate coping strategies are major determinants of patient delay in acute myocardial infarction. *Zeitschrift für Kardiologie*, 91(2): 147–55.

Kenyon, G.M. and Randall, W.L. (2001) Narrative gerontology: an overview. In G. Kenyon, P. Clark, and B. de Vries (eds) *Narrative Gerontology: Theory, Research, and Practice.* New York: Springer.

Kiecolt-Glaser, J.K., McGuire, L., Robles, T.F. and Glaser, R. (2002) Psychoneuroim-munology: psychological influences on immune function and health. *Journal of Consulting and Clinical Psychology*, 70(3): 537–47.

Kivimäki, M., Elovainio, M., Kokko, K., Pulkkinen, L., Kortteinen, M., and Tuomiko-ski, H. (2003) Hostility, unemployment and health status: Testing three theoretical models. *Social Science and Medicine*, 56(10): 2139–52.

Klaus, H.M. and Kennell, J.H. (1976) *Maternal-Infant Bonding.* St. Louis, MO: Mosby.

Kleinhesselink, R.R. and Edwards, R.E. (1975) Seeking and avoiding belief-discrepant information as a function of its perceived refutability. *Journal of Personality and Social Psychology*, 31: 787–90.

Kleinman, A. (1988) *The Illness Narratives: Suffering, Healing and the Human Condition.* New York: Basic Books.

Kobasa, S.C. (1979) Stressful life events, personality and health: an inquiry into hardiness. *Journal of Personality and Social Psychology*, 37: 1–11.

Kohlberg, L. (1969) Stage and sequence: the cognitive-developmental approach to socialization. In D.A. Goslin (ed.) *Handbook of Socialization Theory and Research.* Skokie, IL: Rand McNally.

Kotses, H. and Harver, A. (eds) (1998) *Self-management of Asthma.* New York: Marcel Dekker.

Kübler-Ross, E. (1969) *On Death and Dying.* London: Tavistock/Routledge.

Latané, B. and Darley, J.M. (1968) Group inhibition of bystander intervention in emergencies. *Journal of Personality and Social Psychology*, 10: 215–21.

Lau, R.R. and Hartman, K.A. (1983) Common sense representations of common illness. *Health Psychology*, 2: 319–32.

Lazarus, R.S. (1966) *Psychological Stress and the Coping Process.* New York: McGraw-Hill

Lazarus, R.S. and Averill, J.R. (1972) Emotion and cognition: with special reference to anxiety. In C.D. Spielberger (ed.) *Anxiety: Current Trends in Therapy and Research Volume II.* New York: Academic Press, pp. 241–60.

Lazarus, R.S. and Folkman, S. (1984) *Stress, Appraisal and Coping.* New York: Springer-Verlag.

Leavell, H.R. and Clark, H.G. (1965). *Preventive Medicine for the Doctor in his Community: An Epidemiological Approach*, 3rd edition. New York: McGraw-Hill.

LeFort, S.M., Gray-Donald, K., Rowat, K.M. and Jeans, M.E. (1998) Randomized controlled trial of a community-based psychoeducation program for the self-management of chronic pain. *Pain*, 74(2–3): 297–306.

Lefebvre, J.C., Keefe, F.J., Affleck, G., Raezer, L.B., Starr, K., Caldwell, D.S. and Tennen, H. (1999) The relationship of arthritis self-efficacy to daily pain, daily mood, and daily pain coping in rheumatoid arthritis patients. *Pain*, 80: 425–35.

Levenson, H. (1974) Activism and powerful others: distinctions within the concept of internal–external control. *Journal of Personality Assessment*, 38: 377–83.

Leventhal, H. and Nerenz, D. (1982) Representations of threat and the control of stress. In D. Meichenbaum and J. Jaremki (eds) *Stress Management and Presention: A Cognitive-Behavioural Approach.* New York: Plenum Press.

Levin, J. (2003) Spiritual determinants of health and healing: An epidemiologic perspective on salutogenic mechanisms. *Alternative Therapies in Health and Medicine*, 9(6): 48–57.

Levinson, D.J., Darrow, D.N., Klein, E.B., Levinson, M.H. and McKee, B. (1978) *The Seasons of a Man's Life.* New York: A.A. Knopf.

Lewinsohn, P.M. (1974) A behavioural approach to depression. In R.J. Freidman and M.M. Katz (eds) *The Psychology of Depression: Contemporary Theory and Research.* Washington DC: V.H. Winston, pp. 157–86.

Ley, P. (1997) *Communicating with Patients: Improving Satisfaction and Compliance.* Cheltenham: Stanley Thornes.

Lindblad, A.K., Ring, L., Glimelius, B. and Hansson, M.G. (2002) Focus on the individual – quality of life assessments in oncology. *Acta Oncologica*, 41(6): 507–16.

Linville, P.W. (1987) Self-complexity as a cognitive buffer against stress-related illness and depression. *Journal of Personality and Social Psychology*, 52(4): 663–76.

Lorig, K., Mazanson, P.D. and Holman, H.R. (1993) Evidence suggesting that health education for self-management in patients with chronic arthritis has sustained health benefits while reducing health costs. *Arthritis and Rheumatism*, 36(4): 439–46.

Lund, M.L. and Tamm, M. (2001) How a group of disabled persons experience rehabilitation over a period of time. *Scandinavian Journal of Occupational Therapy*, 8(2): 96–104.

Maccoby, E.E. (1980) *Social Development: Psychological Growth and the Parent-Child Relationship*. New York: Harcourt Brace Jovanovich.

Maddux, J.E. (1993) Social cognitive models of health and exercise behavior: An introduction and review of conceptual issues. *Journal of Applied Sport Psychology*, 5(2): 116–40.

Marks, D.F., Murray, M., Evans, B. and Willig, C. (2000) *Health Psychology: Theory, Research and Practice*. London: Sage.

Marmot, M., Siegrist, J., Theorell, T. and Feeney, A. (1999) Health and the psychosocial environment at work. In M. Marmot and R.G. Wilkinson (eds) *Social Determinants of Health*. Oxford: Oxford University Press, pp. 105–31.

Marsland, A.L., Bachen, E.A., Cohen, S., Rabin, B. and Manuck, S.B. (2002) Stress, immune reactivity and susceptibility to infectious disease. *Physiology and Behaviour*, 77: 711–16.

Maslow, A.H. (1970) *Motivation and Personality*, 2nd edition. New York: Harper & Row

Matthews, S., Stansfield, S. and Power, C. (1999) Social support at age 33: The influence of gender, employment status and social class. *Social Science and Medicine*, 49: 133–42.

McGaugh, J.L. (2003) *Memory and Emotion: The Making of Lasting Memories*. New York: Columbia University Press.

McGrath, J.E. (1970) A conceptual formulation for research on stress. In J.E. McGrath (ed.) *Social and Psychological Factors in Stress*. New York: Holt, Rinehart & Winston, pp. 10–21.

Meadows, S. (1993) *The Child as Thinker*. London: Routledge.

Michie, S., French, D., Allanson, A., Bobrow, M., Marteau, T.M. (1997) Information recall in genetic counselling: a pilot study of its assessment. *Patient Education and Counseling*, 32(1–2): 93–100.

Miller, G.A. (1956) The magical number seven, plus or minus two: some limits to our capacity for processing information. *Psychological Review*, 63: 81–97.

Miller, J.F. (1992) Analysis of coping with illness. In J.F. Miller (ed.) *Coping with Chronic Illness: Overcoming Powerlessness*, 2nd edition. Philadelphia: F.A. Davis, pp. 19–49.

Mills, M. and Walker, J.M. (1994) Memory, mood and dementia. *Journal of Aging Studies*, 8(1): 17–27.

Mirowsky, J. and Ross, C. (2003) *Social Causes of Psychological Distress*, 2nd edition. New York: Aldine de Gruyter.

Morley, S., Eccleston, C. and Williams, A. (1999) Systematic review and meta-analysis of randomized controlled trials of cognitive behaviour therapy and behaviour therapy for chronic pain in adults, excluding headache. *Pain*, 80: 1–13.

Morris, J. and Ingham, R. (1988) Choice of surgery for early breast cancer: psychosocial considerations. *Social Science and Medicine*, 27(11): 1257–62.

Muntner, P. Sudre, P., Uldry, C., Rochat, T., Courteheuse, C., Naef, A.F. and Perneger, T.V. (2001) Predictors of participation and attendance in a new asthma patient self-management education program. *Chest*, 120(3): 778–84.

Murray, M. (2003) Narrative psychology. In J.A. Smith (ed.). *Qualitative Psychology: A Practical Guide to Research Methods*. Thousand Oaks, CA: Sage, pp. 111–31.

Newell, R. (2002a) Living with disfigurement. *Nursing Times*, 98(15): 34–5.

Newell, R. (2002b) The fear-avoidance model: Helping patients to cope with disfigurement. *Nursing Times*, 98(16): 38–9.

Nicholas, P.K. (1993) Hardiness, self-care practices and perceived health status in older adults. *Journal of Advanced Nursing*, 18(7): 1085–94.

Norman, P. and Bennett, P. (1995) Health locus of control. In Conner M. and Norman P. (eds) *Predicting health behaviour*. Buckingham: Open University Press.

O'Boyle, C.A., McGee, H.N., Hickey, A. *et al.* (1993) *The Schedule for the Evaluation of Individual Quality of Life (SEIQoL): Administration Manual.* Dublin: Department of Psychology, Royal College of Surgeons in Ireland.

O'Connell, K., Skevington, S. and Saxena, S. (2003) Preliminary development of the World Health Organsiation's Quality of Life HIV instrument (WHOQOL-HIV): analysis of the pilot version. *Social Science and Medicine*, 57(7): 1259–75.

Omoto, A.M. and Snyder, M. (1995) Sustained helping without obligation: Motivation, longevity of service, and perceived attitude change among AIDS volunteers. *Journal of Personality and Social Psychology*, 68(4): 671–86.

Osiri, M., Welch, V., Brosseau, L., Shea, B., McGowan, J., Tugwell, P. and Wells, G. (2003) Transcutaneous electrical nerve stimulation for knee osteoarthritis (Cochrane Review). In *The Cochrane Library* 4. Chichester: Wiley.

Overmier, J.B. and Murison, R. (2000) Anxiety and helplessness in the face of stress predisposes, precipitates and sustains gastric ulceration. *Behavioural Brain Research*, 110: 161–74.

Paley, G. and Shapiro, D.A. (2002) Lessons from psychotherapy research for psychological interventions for people with schizophrenia. *Psychology and Psychotherapy: Theory, Research and Practice*, 75(1): 5–17.

Park, C.L., Folkman, S. and Bostrom, A. (2001) Appraisals of controllability and coping in caregivers and HIV+ men: Testing the goodness-of-fit hypothesis. *Journal of Consulting and Clinical Psychology*, 69(3): 481–8.

Park, D.C., Hertzog, C., Leventhal, H., Morrell, R.W., Leventhal, E., Birchmore, D., Martin, M. and Bennett J. (1999) Medication adherence in rheumatoid arthritis patients: older is wiser (comments). *Journal of the American Geriatrics Society*, 48(4): 457–9.

Parker, G., Roy, K. and Eyers, K. (2003) Cognitive behavior therapy for depression? Choose horses for courses. *American Journal of Psychiatry*, 160(5): 825–34.

Parkes, C.M. (1975) *Bereavement – Studies of Grief in Adult Life.* Harmondsworth: Penguin.

Paterson C. (2003) MYMOP2. http://www.hsrc.ac.uk/mymop/entrymymop.htm

Payne, S.A., Dean, S.J. and Kalus, C. (1998) A comparative study of death anxiety in hospice and emergency nurses. *Journal of Advanced Nursing*, 28(4): 700–6.

Pennebaker, J.W. (1993) Putting stress into words: Health, linguistic and therapeutic implications. *Behavior Research and Therapy*, 31(6): 539–48.

Pennebaker, J.W. and Seagal, J.D. (1999) Forming a story: The health benefits of narrative. *Journal of Clinical Psychology*, 55(10): 1243–54.

Peters, M.L., Godaert, G.L.R., Balliieux, R.E., Brosschot, J.F., Sweep, F.C.G.J. *et al.* (1999) Immune response to experimental stress: Effects of mental effort and uncontrollability. *Psychosomatic Medicine*, 61: 513–24.

Petty, R.E. and Cacioppo, J.T. (1986) *Communication and Persuasion: Central and Peripheral Routes to Attitude Change.* New York: Springer-Verlag.

Piaget, J. (1929) *The Child's Concept of the World.* London: Routledge & Kegan Paul.

Piaget, J. (1951) *Play, Dreams and Imitation in Children.* London: Routledge & Kegan Paul.

Piaget, J. (1963) *The Origins of Intelligence in Children.* New York: Norton.

Piaget, J. and Inhelder, B. (1956) *The Child's Conception of Space.* London: Routledge & Kegan Paul.

Price, B. (1990) *Body Image: Nursing Concepts and Care.* New York: Prentice Hall.

Price, J.R. and Couper, J. (2003) Cognitive behaviour therapy for chronic fatigue syndrome in adults (Cochrane Review). In *The Cochrane Library* 4. Chichester: Wiley.

Prochaska, J.O. and DiClemente, C.C. (1983) Stages and processes of self change in smoking: Towards an integrative model of change. *Journal of Consulting and Clinical Psychology*, 51: 390–5.

Purdie, N. and McCrindle, A. (2002) Self-regulation, self-efficacy and health behavior change in older adults. *Educational Gerontology*, 28(5): 379–400.

Radley, A. (1994) *Making Sense of Illness: The Social Psychology of Health and Disease.* London: Sage.

Reason, J. (1990) *Human Error.* Cambridge: Cambridge University Press.

Rief, W., Ihle, D. and Pilger, F. (2003) A new approach to assess illness behaviour. *Journal of Psychosomatic Research*, 54(5): 415–16.

Riemsma, R.P., Pattenden, J., Bridle, C., Sowden, A.J., Mather, L., Watt, I.S. and Walker, A. (2003) Systematic review of the effectiveness of stage based interventions to promote smoking cessation. *British Medical Journal*, 326(7400): 1175–7.

Robertson, J. and Robertson J. (1967–73) Young children in brief separation (videos). http://www.childdevmedia.com/

Rose, S., Bisson, J. and Wessely, S. (2004) Psychological debriefing for preventing post traumatic stress disorder (PTSD) (Cochrane Review). In *The Cochrane Library*, 1. Chichester: Wiley.

Rosenhan, D.L. (1973) On being sane in insane places. *Science*, 179: 365–9.

Rosenstiel, A.K. and Keefe, F.J. (1983) The use of coping strategies in chronic low back pain patients: Relationship to patient characteristics and current adjustment. *Pain*, 17: 33–44.

Rosenstock, I.M. (1974a) Historical origins of the health belief model. *Health Education Monographs*, 2: 328–35.

Rosenstock, I.M. (1974b) The health belief model and preventive health behaviour. *Health Education Monographs*, 2: 354–86.

Rosenstock, I.M., Strecher, V.J. and Becker, M.H. (1988) Social learning theory and the health belief model. *Health Education Quarterly*, 15: 175–83.

Rosenthal, R. and Jacobson, L. (1968) *Pygmalion in the Classroom: Teacher Expectations and Pupils' Intellectual Development.* New York: Holt, Rinehart and Winston.

Ross, C.E. and Mirowsky, J. (1989) Explaining the social patterns of depression: Control and problem solving – or support and talking? *Journal of Health and Social Behavior*, 30(2): 206–19.

Rotter, J.B. (1966) Generalized expectancies for internal versus external control of reinforcement. *Psychological Monographs: General and Applied*, 80(1): 1–28.

Rubin, M. and Hewstone, M. (1998) Social identity theory's self-esteem hypothesis: A review and some suggestions for clarification. *Personality and Social Psychology Review*, 2(1): 40–62.

Rushforth, H. (1999) Practitioner review: communicating with hospitalized children: review and application of research pertaining to children's understanding of health and illness. *Journal of Child Psychology and Psychiatry*, 40(5): 683–91.

Rutter, M. (1979) Maternal deprivation, 1972–1978: New findings, new concepts, new approaches. *Child Development*, 50: 282–305.

Sanders-Dewey, N.E.J., Mullins, L.L. and Chaney, J.M. (2001) Coping style, perceived uncertainty in illness, and distress in individuals with Parkinson's disease and their caregivers. *Rehabilitation Psychology*, 46(4): 363–81.

Sanz, E.J. (2003) Concordance and children's use of medicines. *British Medical Journal*, 327(7419): 858–60.

Schaffer, D.R. (1988) *Social and Personality Development*, 2nd edition. Pacific Grove, CA: Brooks Cole.

Seligman M.E.P. (1975) *Helplessness: On Development, Depression and Death.* New York: Freeman.

Seligman, M.E.P. and Maier, S.F. (1967) Failure to escape traumatic shock. *Journal of Experimental Psychology*, 74: 1–9.

Seligman, M.E.P., Maier, S.F. and Geer, J.H. (1968) Alleviation of learned helplessness in the dog. *Journal of Abnormal Psychology*, 88(3): 242–7.

Selye, H. (1956) *The Stress of Life.* New York: McGraw-Hill.

Sephton, S.E., Koopman, C., Schaal, M., Thorsens, C. and Spiegel, D. (2001) Spiritual expression and immune status in women with metastic breast cancer: an exploratory study. *The Breast Journal*, 7(5): 345–53.

Sheeran, P. and Abraham, C. (1996) The health belief model. In M. Conner and P. Norman (eds), *Predicting Health Behaviour: Research and Practice with Social Cognition Models*. Buckingham: Open University Press, pp. 23–61.

Sherman, D.W. (1996) Nurses' willingness to care for AIDS patients and spirituality, social support, and death anxiety. *Image – the Journal of Nursing Scholarship*, 28(3): 205–13.

Skevington, S.M., Bradshaw, J. and Saxena, S. (1999) Selecting national items for the WHOQOL: Conceptual and psychometric considerations. *Social Science and Medicine*, 48(4): 473–87.

Sliwinski, M.J., Hofer, S.M., Hall, C., Buschke, H. and Lipton, R.B. (2003) Modeling memory decline in older adults: The importance of preclinical dementia, attrition, and chronological age. *Psychology and Aging*, 18(4): 658–671.

Snyder, C.R. (1998) A case for hope in pain, loss and suffering. In J.H. Harvey (ed.) *Perspectives on Loss: A Sourcebook*. Philadelphia: Brunner Mazel.

Spieker, S.J. and Bensley, L. (1994) Roles of living arrangements and grandmother social support in adolescent mothering and infant attachment. *Developmental Psychology*, 30(1): 102–11.

Srivastava, S., John, O.P., Gosling, S.D. and Potter, J. (2003) Development of personality in early and middle adulthood: Set like plaster or persistent change? *Journal of Personality and Social Psychology*, 84(5): 1041–53.

Stansfield, S.A. (1999) Social support and social cohesion. In M. Marmot and R.G. Wilkinson (eds) *Social Determinants of Health*. Oxford: Oxford University Press, pp. 155–78.

Stewart, K. (2002) *Helping a Child with Nonverbal Learning Disorder or Asperger's Syndrome: A Parent's Guide*. Oakland, CA: New Harbinger Publications.

Stockwell, F. (1984) *The Unpopular Patient*. London: Croom Helm.

Stroebe, M.S. and Schut, H. (1998) Culture and grief. *Bereavement Care*, 17(1): 7–10.

Stroebe, W. and Stroebe, M.S. (1987) *Bereavement and Health: The Psychological and Physical Consequences of Partner Loss*. New York: Cambridge University Press.

Tajfel, H. (1982) *Social Identity and Intergroup Relations*. Cambridge: Cambridge University Press.

Taris, T.W. and Bok, I.A. (1996) Effects of parenting style upon psychological well-being of young adults: Exploring the relations among parental care, locus of control and depression. *Early Child Development and Care*, 132: 93–104.

Taylor, S.E. (1979) Patient hospital behaviour: Reactance, helplessness, or control? *Journal of Social Issues*, 35: 156–84.

Taylor, S.E. and Brown, J.D. (1988) Illusion and well-being: A social psychological perspective on mental health. *Psychological Bulletin*, 103(2): 193–210.

Taylor, S.E. and Gollwitzer, P.M. (1995) Effects of mindset on positive illusions. *Journal of Personality and Social Psychology*, 69: 213–26.

Tedstone, J.E. and Tarrier, N. (2003) Posttraumatic stress disorder following medical illness and treatment. *Clinical Psychology Review*, 23: 409–48.

Temoshok, L. (1987) Personality, coping style, emotion and cancer: Towards an integrative model. *Cancer Surveys*, 6(iii): 545–67.

Teresi, J.A., Holmes, D. Ramirez, M. Gurland, B.J. and Lantigua, R. (2001) Performance of cognitive tests among different racial/ethnic and education groups: Findings of differential item functioning and possible item bias. *Journal of Mental Health and Aging*, 7(1): 79–89.

Toth, E.L., Majumdar, S.R., Guirguis, L.M., Lewanczuk, R.Z., Lee, T.K. and Johnson, J.A. (2003) Compliance with clinical practice guidelines for type 2 diabetes in rural patients: Treatment gaps and opportunities for improvement. *Pharmacotherapy*, 23(5): 659–65.

Uchino, B.N., Cacioppo, J.T. and Kiecolt-Glaser, J.K. (1996) The relationship between social support and physiological processes: A review with emphasis on underlying mechanisms and implications for health. *Psychological Bulletin*, 119(3): 488–531.

Vachon, M.L., Sheldon, A.R., Lancee, W.J., Lyall, W.A., Rogers, J. and Freeman, S.J. (1982) Correlates of enduring distress patterns following bereavement: Social network, life situation and personality. *Psychological Medicine*, 12(4): 783–8.

Van Doorn, C., Kasl, S.V., Beery, L.C., Jacobs, S.C. and Prigerson, H.G. (1998) The influence of marital quality and attachment styles on traumatic grief and depressive symptoms. *Journal of Nervous and Mental Disease*, 186(9): 566–73.

van Tulder, M.W., Ostelo, R.W.J.G., Vlaeyen, J.W.S., Linton, S.J., Morley, S.J. and Assendelft, W.J.J. (2003) Behavioural treatment for chronic low back pain (Cochrane Review). In *The Cochrane Library* 4. Chichester: Wiley.

Vedhara, K., McDermott, M.P., Evans, T.G., Treanor, J.J., Plummer, S. *et al.* (2002) Chronic stress in nonelderly caregivers: psychological, endocrine and immune implications. *Journal of Psychosomatic Research*, 53: 1153–61.

Veldtman, G.R., Matley, S.L., Kendall, L., Quirk, J., Gibbs, J.L., Parsons, J.M. and Hewison J. (2000) Illness understanding in children and adolescents with heart disease. *Heart*, 84(4): 395–7.

Vlaeyen, J.W.S. and Linton, S.J. (2000) Fear-avoidance and its consequences in chronic musculoskeletal pain: a state of the art. *Pain*, 85: 3127–332.

Vollrath, M. and Torgersen, S. (2000) Personality types and coping. *Personality and Individual Differences*, 29(2): 367–78.

Von Korff, M., Moore, J.E., Lorig, K., Cherkin, D.C., Saunders, K., Gonzalez, V.M., Laurent, D., Rutter, C. and Comite, F. (1998) A randomized trial of a lay person-led self-management group intervention for back pain patients in primary care. *Spine*, 23(23): 2608–15.

Vygotsky, L.S. (1978) *Mind in Society: The Development of Higher Mental Processes*. Cambridge, MA: Harvard University Press.

Walker, J.M. (1989) The nursing management of pain in the elderly. Unpublished PhD thesis, Dorset Institute (Bournemouth University).

Walker, J.M. (1993) A social behavioural approach to understanding and promoting condom use. In J. Wilson-Barnett and J. Macleod Clark (eds) *Research in Health Promotion and Nursing*. Basingstoke: Macmillan.

Walker, J. (2001) *Control and the Psychology of Health*. Buckingham: Open University Press.

Walker, J. and Sofaer, B. (1998) Predictors of psychological distress in chronic pain patients. *Journal of Advanced Nursing*, 27: 320–6.

Walker, J.M., Akinsanya, J.A., Davis, B. and Marcer, D. (1990) The nursing management of elderly patients with pain in the community: study and recommendations. *Journal of Advanced Nursing*, 15: 1154–61.

Walker, J., Brooksby, A., McInerny, J. and Taylor, A. (1998) Patients' judgements about hospital care: Building confidence and trust. *Journal of Nursing Management*, 6: 193–200.

Walker, J., Holloway, I. and Sofaer, B. (1999) 'In the system': patients' experiences of chronic back pain. *Pain*, 80: 621–8

Wallhagen, M.I., Strawbridge, W.J., Kaplan, G.A. and Cohen, R.D. (1994) Impact of internal health locus of control on health outcomes for older men and women: A longitudinal perspective. *Gerontologist*, 34(3): 299–306.

Wallston, K.A. (1992) Hocus pocus, the focus isn't strictly on locus: Rotter's social learning theory modified for health. *Cognitive Theory and Research*, 16(2): 183–99.

Wallston, K.A., Wallston, B.S. and DeVellis, R. (1978) Development of the Multidimensional Health Locus of Control (MHLOC) scale. *Health Education Monographs*, 6: 161–70.

Walter, T. (1996) *The Revival of Death*. London: Routledge.

Weinman, J., Petrie, K.J., Sharpe, N. and Walker, S. (2004) The Illness Perception Questionnaire. www.uib.no/ipq/

Wiebe, D.J. and Korbel, C. (2003) Defensive denial, self-regulation and health. In L.D. Cameron and H. Leventhal (eds) *The Self-regulation of Health and Illness Behaviour*. London: Routledge.

Witte, K. and Allen, M. (2000) A meta-analysis of fear appeals: Implications for effective public health campaigns. *Health Education and Behavior*, 27(5): 591–615.

Wolpe, J. (1958) *Psychotherapy by Reciprocal Inhibition*. Stanford, CA: Stanford University Press.

World Health Organisation (2004a) Definition of health. www.who.int/about/ definition/en/

World Health Organization (2004b) WHOQOL: measuring quality of life. http:// www.who.int/evidence/assessment-instruments/qol/

World Health Organization (2001) *The World Health Report 2001*. Mental health: new understanding, new hope. www.who.int/whr2001/2001/main/en/chapter3/ 003d.htm

Wortman, C.B. and Silver, R.C. (1989) The myths of coping with loss. *Journal of Consulting and Clinical Psychology*, 57(3): 349–57.

Zborowski, M. (1969) *People in Pain*. San Francisco: Jossey-Bass.

INDEX

Page numbers in *italics* refer to tables and figures.

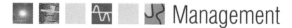
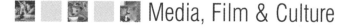
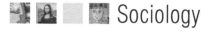
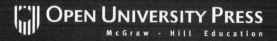
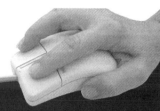